IMAGES
of America

DANVERS STATE HOSPITAL

On the Cover: This is a vintage postcard of Danvers State Hospital (DSH) in the 1930s. (John Gray.)

IMAGES
of America

DANVERS STATE HOSPITAL

Katherine Anderson and Robert Duffy
Introduction by John Archer

ARCADIA
PUBLISHING

ISBN 978-1-4671-2766-0

Published by Arcadia Publishing
Charleston, South Carolina

Printed in the United States of America

Library of Congress Control Number: 2017942406

For all general information, please contact Arcadia Publishing:
Telephone 843-853-2070
Fax 843-853-0044
E-mail sales@arcadiapublishing.com
For customer service and orders:
Toll-Free 1-888-313-2665

Visit us on the Internet at www.arcadiapublishing.com

To all who called Danvers State Hospital home. To those who fought to save the hospital, and those who continue the fight to memorialize it.

Contents

ACKNOWLEDGMENTS

As historians, we frequently lament the short amount of time we have to document the buildings that speak to us in a unique and powerful way. Danvers is certainly one of these, resonating with us long after its demolition. This book would not have been possible without the help of those who keep the memories of Danvers State alive.

Our greatest debt of gratitude is given to John Archer, the "King of the Kirkbride," who welcomed us into his home and trusted us with his collection. We are also indebted to Richard Trask, archivist at the Peabody Institute Library, who provided us with a number of rare historic images. Many thanks as well to the staff at the Massachusetts Archives who worked to locate every last piece of Danvers history. The completion of this book also relied heavily on John Gray and his expansive collection of photographs, both historical and his own incredible body of work. We also extend our thanks to the photographers and collectors who graciously shared their collections: Karen Bourdelais, David Walsh, Amanda Kohut, Ben Kenny, Daniel Runyan, Ethan Dexter, Jett Chapman, and John Duffill, as well as to Marcia Cini for the use of her graduate thesis.

Danvers State Hospital was, in the end, far more than just the haunted castle on the hill where teenagers dared one another to enter. The asylum on the hill was an integral part of the fabric of mental health history, a model institution where medical advances were made daily in the treatment of mental illness. In the end, the state hospital would descend into the annals of history as a "snake pit" of death and despair, tales of neglect and abuse eclipsing the accomplishments of its early years.

The very public fight for the Kirkbride reminded the public of what the asylum was meant to be, an institution offering shelter and healing for those with mental illness, a place of transformational care where memories were made and minds were healed. This book was conceived with the hope that Danvers might live on and the very important conversation about mental health care will continue.

INTRODUCTION

> *I come to present the strong claims of suffering humanity . . . the condition of the miserable, the desolate, the outcast. I come as the advocate of the helpless, forgotten insane men and women; of beings sunk to a condition from which the unconcerned world would start with real horror.*
>
> —Dorothea Dix, from her memorial to the Massachusetts Legislature

From the moment the modern asylum was first conceived in the United States, there was a need for reform. Many asylums filled their wards before their doors were even officially opened, taking transfers from local prisons and almshouses. The number of mentally ill in the nation seemed to grow overnight, and most states were ill prepared to take on such a plight. It was clear that improvements were necessary.

In 1841, Boston school teacher Dorothea Dix was asked to teach a Sunday school class at a jail in Cambridge. While there, Dix discovered that mentally ill women were confined together with criminals in filthy cells with no heat. She would come to find that this was the case in nearly every institution in the state where the jails and poorhouses were largely unregulated and underfunded, resulting in widespread abuse. Dix published her findings and presented them to the Massachusetts State Legislature. Her passion would ignite a wave of reform that resulted in a bill to expand the state's mental hospital at Worcester.

Nearly 30 years later, the state authorized the building of a fourth asylum at Danvers (formerly Salem) to alleviate the overcrowding at Worcester, Taunton, and Northampton. In the midst of a depression that would end shortly after the opening of the hospital, then-governor of Massachusetts Alexander H. Rice approved the plans to build the new asylum on Hathorne Hill. The site was chosen not just for its beauty and spectacular views, but also for its isolation from the day to day hustle of the Bay State. The first group of hospital trustees believed firmly that the hospital would be a model of care, one of curative value as opposed to custodial. It was their hope that, through advances in modern medicine and high-quality education, that those patients entering into the asylum, would find a temporary home where they might get well and return as contributing members to their families.

Despite numerous reservations about the cost of the asylum on the hill, the state continued to allocate money for the completion of the project. A reservoir was dug, a water and sewage system installed. Roads were cut into the hillside and brick was laid. From the sky, Danvers resembled a bat with its wings outstretched, the stepped back wards flanking a central administration building. Red Danvers brick and granite mined in Massachusetts graced the grand façade, the towers topped with wrought iron crowns decorated with dahlias—the Victorian symbol for madness.

In their first annual report, the trustees wrote:

> The State has an institution with every modern improvement; and the Trustees, assisted by the Superintendent, are endeavoring to make it a model institution, having in view a hospital for the cure of patients, rather than an asylum for the chronic insane...The Hospital having been in operation but a short time, the Trustees necessarily have limited experience and knowledge of its working capacities for the great objects of charity and humanity for which it was designed and built; yet, with that limited experience and knowledge, they concur in the belief that, when in full operation, it will rank among the most useful of the charitable institutions in the Commonwealth.

Though Danvers would eventually succumb to the same ills as most institutions for the care of the mentally ill in the United States, it serves as far more than just an icon of the mid-century madhouse. It was more than just the stuff of urban legend, fodder for ghost stories, and childish dares. There is another side to asylums, a dark past that was first painted with the bright light of hope.

Dr. Thomas Story Kirkbride was a visionary who sought to offer holistic treatment for those who suffered from various types of mental illness, which could have been as simple as teen-aged angst, a quick temper, or simply a penchant for a bit more independence of thought than was acceptable in the late-19th century. Kirkbride's vision, so ahead of his time, offered fresh country air, manageable sizes for treatment wards, walks in the country sunshine, and simple gardening activities for the patients so that they could help to grow some of their own food, and flowers for the wards. The surroundings were designed to be not just functional, but beautiful, with classic proportions, beautiful woodwork, and soothing landscaping. Kirkbride sought to create a space that would be "curative, not custodial," which was a radical notion in his day. Most people thought the mentally ill should be locked away in nothing better than a prison but Kirkbride knew better.

Being a Quaker, Kirkbride believed that those suffering from mental illness should be cared for with the same empathetic dedication as those afflicted with a common physical ailment. He reminded his fellow asylum doctors that their patients were human beings, not numbers (as so many became when they died on the premises and were interred only by a number marker in the cemetery on the hill, just like the one on Hathorne Hill, where Danvers State Hospital was located). "There is no reason," Kirkbride wrote, "why an individual, who has the misfortune to become insane, should, on that account, be deprived of any comfort or even luxury." Not only were we meant to strive to find understanding; we were meant to care for the mentally ill and want the best for them—a cure for madness.

This, after all, is the point of hospitals, is it not? That people who enter while ill will leave again, restored to good health. The abuses and horrors that happened in the mid-20th century at Danvers State and other mental health institutions came about through poor fiduciary management and even poorer supervision by the state. Overcrowding led to patient abuses and neglect, and by the late 20th century, most of these institutions became the objects of urban legends or playgrounds for urban explorers.

In the early-20th century, asylum superintendents would begin to ignore Kirkbride's tenets of moral treatment in favor of cost cutting measures. With the advent of drug therapies, the hospital's maximum capacity was repeatedly tested with patients being housed in attics, day rooms, and hallways. Kirkbride's vision of individualized care and treatment was no longer feasible, and the asylum structure collapsed into the snake pits of popular culture. Deinstitutionalization would sweep through the asylums, emptying the wards and closing their doors for good.

It is all too easy to forget the good intent with which Thomas Kirkbride developed his theories on the housing and treatment of the mentally ill. It was with the best of intentions that he laid the foundation for Nathaniel Bradlee's "castle on the hill," which stood so proudly, for so long, high above little Danvers town. This "veritable nest of beauty" welcomed neighbors from nearby towns to come and visit the grounds, and provided what was hoped to be a temporary, healing home for its patients.

Eventually, Danvers would become yet another piece of "surplus property" that the State of Massachusetts was eager to unload. The resulting firestorm spanned years with nearly all attempts at preservation shot down by the state and the private developers that would eventually take charge of the "Hospital Palace." As early as the 1980s, it was suggested that much of the Kirkbride could be retained, but in the end, the battle was lost and with it, the history of one of the most influential and forward-thinking asylums of the 19th Century.

Asylums such as Danvers hold rich histories both from a medical standpoint and from a human standpoint. The sheer volume of human history that is contained in a place such as Danvers State Hospital cannot be calculated by those who arrive on the scene long after it has been demolished. As such, however, the state hospital draws a distinct line in the sand, separating those who would remember from those who would prefer to forget. It is, at times, difficult to see the forest for the trees, to remember that those who do not learn from history are doomed to repeat it. The asylum system of the United States is perhaps one of the best representations of that, as we continue to dismantle every last stone and erase every last memory of what once graced one of the highest points in the town of Danvers.

Though Danvers State Hospital no longer exists as it was originally conceived, it remains a substantial part of our present. It is the past, certainly, but it is also the here and now, existing still in the hearts and minds of those who fought for its preservation and those who continue to fight for the memorialization of the hospital. Those who continue to educate others on the treatment of the mentally ill carry the stories of Danvers within them, and it will forever be a monument to our ability (or inability as the case may be) to care for the most vulnerable of our population.

Katherine Anderson and Robert Duffy have a unique passion for these buildings. They imagine what life was like on the wards and strive to tell those stories to the best of their abilities. This book brings it all alive for us with text and photographs that allow us a window into the past, much as H.G. Wells imagined his time machine might do. Will you join me as we travel back in time to those "good old days" in Danvers?

—John Archer

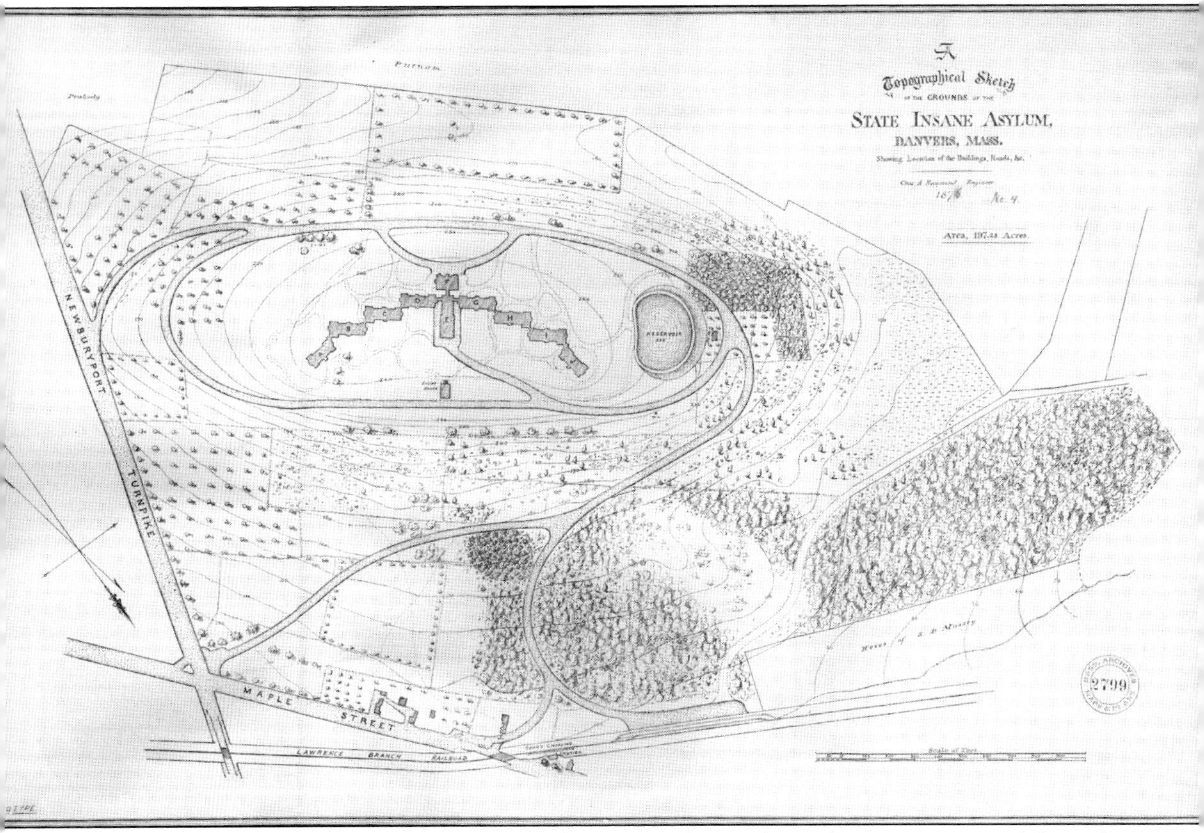

The site on Hathorne Hill, some 257 feet high, was chosen for its location, removed from the congestion of the city with sweeping views from the crest of the hill. The site, originally 197.25 acres, was purchased for $39,542.50. Chosen also for its beauty and privacy, the site lay 18 miles north of Boston and seven miles from the coal port at Salem. The Swan's Crossing station on the Lawrence Branch of the Eastern Railroad lay to the north. This topographical sketch of the grounds dated 1876 shows the location of the main Kirkbride, the reservoir that would be the asylum's main source of water and the roads that would be constructed to connect the hospital with the main thoroughfares of the time. In places, the sketch even details what trees were to be planted on the grounds. (Massachusetts Archives.)

One

Hospital Palace

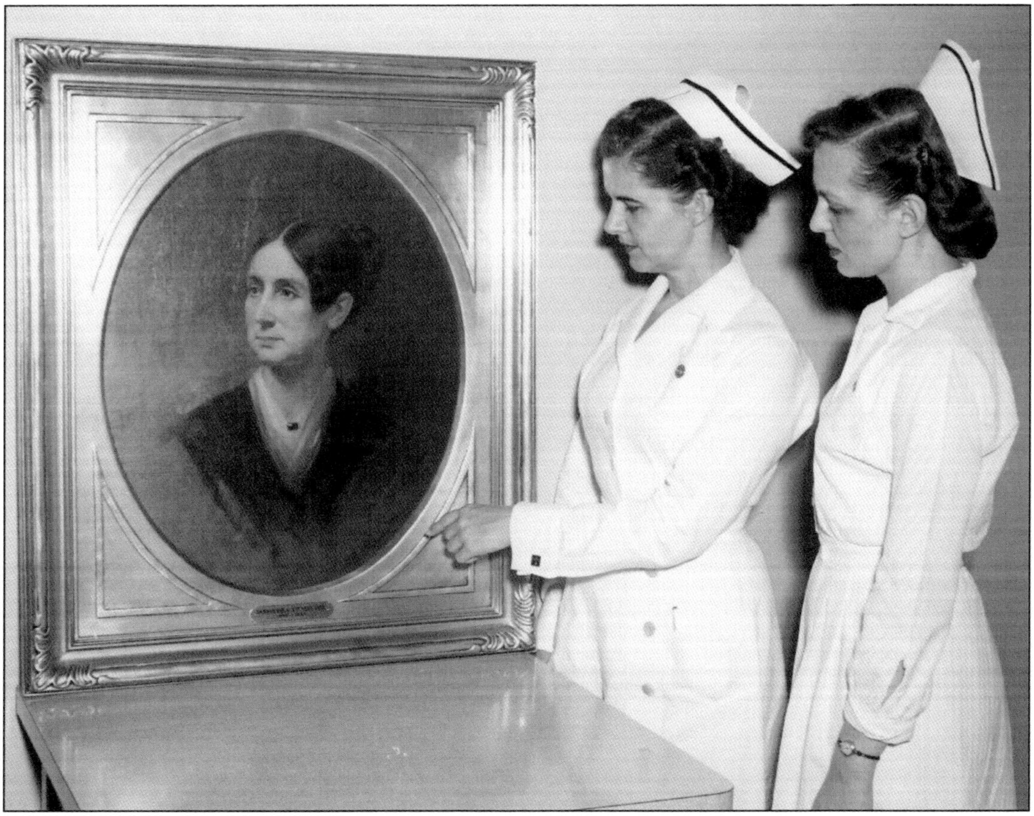

Through the efforts of reformer Dorothea Dix, who presented her memorial to the legislature in 1843, Dix called attention to the state of the insane who were "chained, naked, beaten with rods." Dix was instrumental in the improvement of existing asylum as well as the construction of new ones. She championed the moral treatment of the insane, and her efforts had significant national impact. (US National Library of Medicine.)

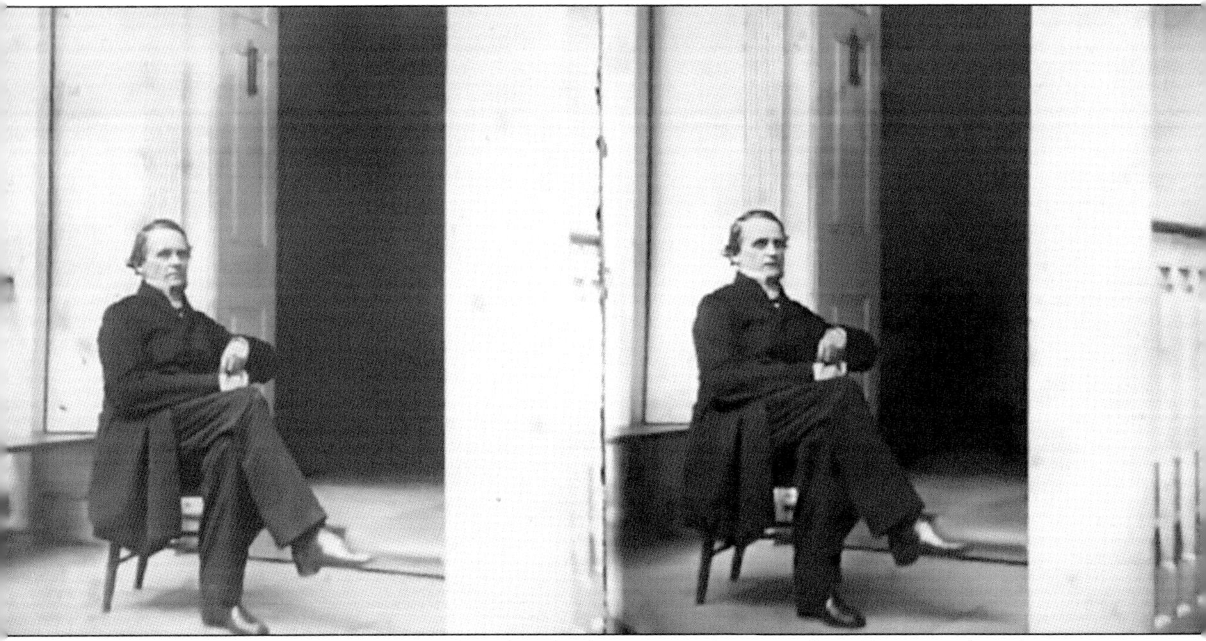

Danvers State Hospital, the fourth asylum built in Massachusetts after Worcester (1832), Taunton (1851), and Northampton (1856), was constructed according to the Kirkbride Plan, developed by Dr. Thomas Story Kirkbride. Kirkbride was the first chief physician of the Pennsylvania Hospital for the Insane and became a strong advocate for the moral treatment for the insane. Patients in hospitals with private patient rooms, grand architectural design, and peaceful natural surroundings. (Robert Duffy.)

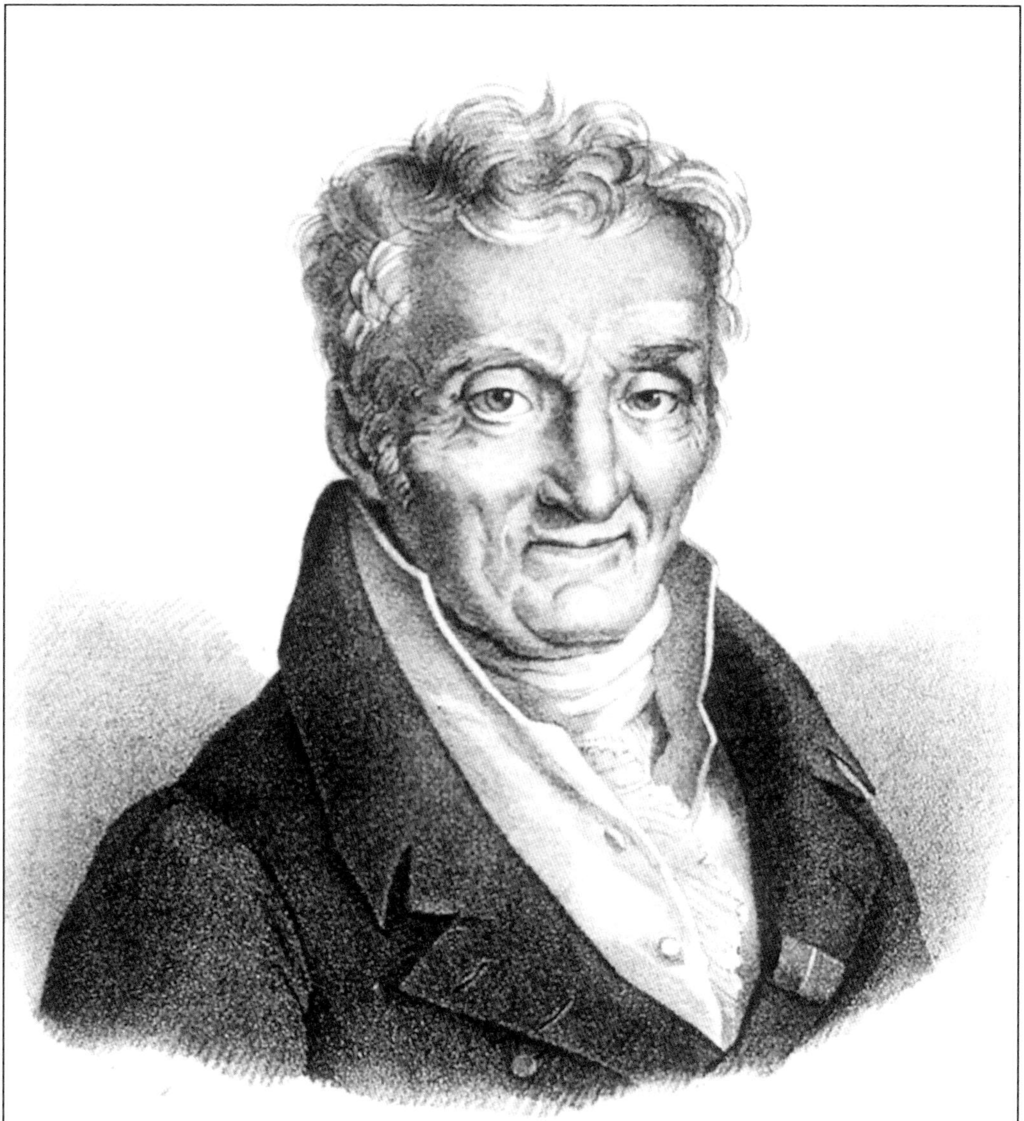

Ten years after Dix presented her memorial to the legislature, Dr. Thomas Story Kirkbride published his treatise *On the Construction, Organization, and General Arrangements of Hospitals for the Insane*, in which he detailed an institutional model that would later become the architectural plan for Danvers State Hospital. The Kirkbride Plan suggested that the asylum be built in the country, on at least 100 acres, while remaining accessible in all seasons. The hospital itself should be composed of eight wards housing a maximum of 250 patients separated by sex, with the most "excited" patients residing in the outermost wings of the wards that flanked the main administration building. Kirkbride's plan was grounded in the belief that the hospital's function was primarily curative rather than custodial; patients were meant to recuperate surrounded by "fresh air and pure water." He believed, as did Philippe Pinel (pictured here) and William Tuke, that the insane needed the same opportunities to get well as those suffering from any other disease. (Robert Duffy.)

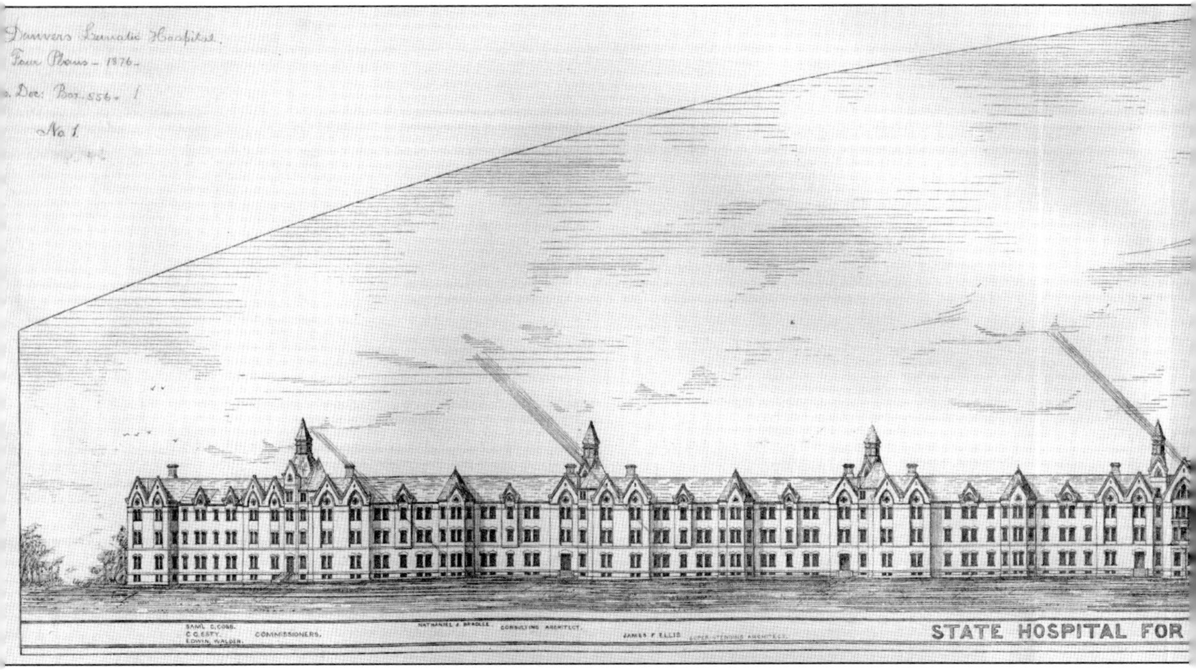

Authorization was given for the construction of the Danvers State Insane Asylum in 1873 and subsequently began on May 1, 1874. The asylums at Worcester, Taunton, and Northampton were already overcrowded, as was the almshouse at Tewksbury. As plans moved forward to

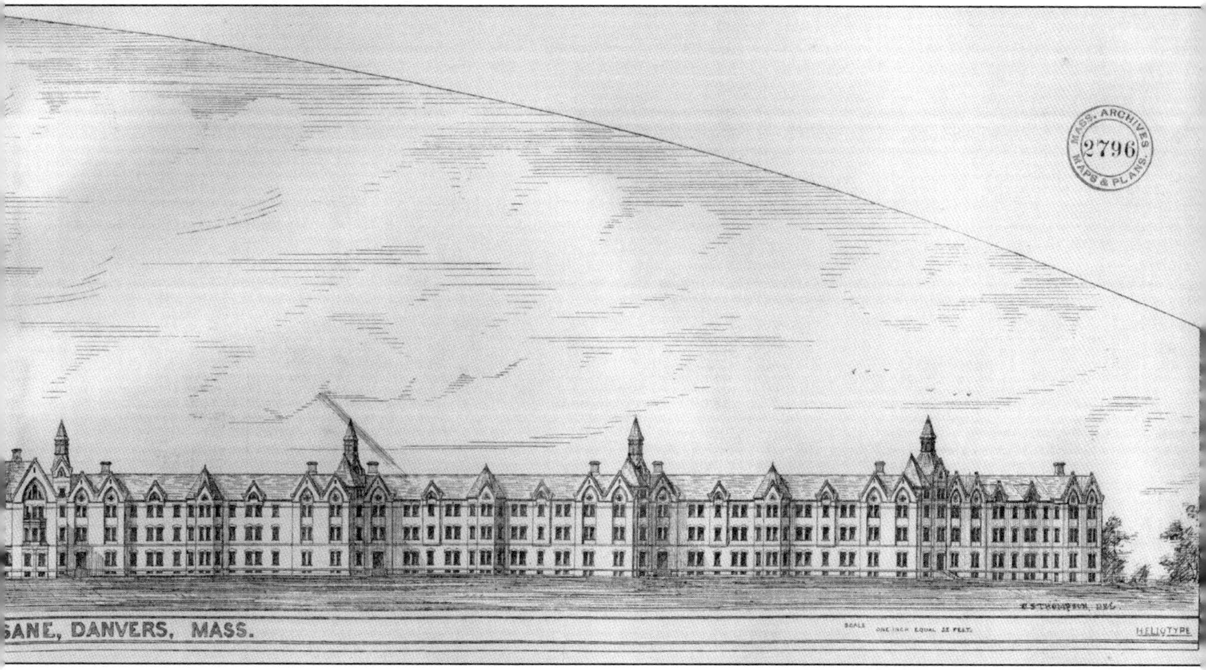

also close the city asylum at South Boston, the Commonwealth chose Danvers as the site for the new asylum to serve primarily Essex County as well as the overflow from South Boston. (Massachusetts Archives.)

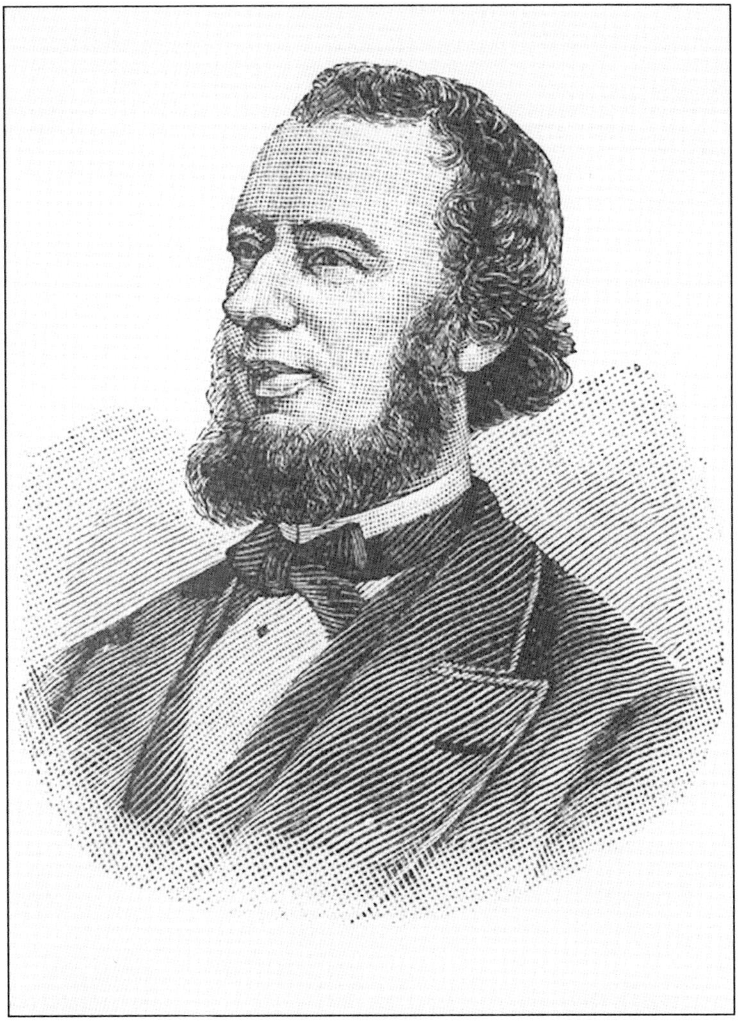

Nearly 200 acres were purchased, and prominent Boston architect Nathaniel J. Bradlee was chosen to design the facility. Bradlee had already established a legacy of landmark buildings in Boston and the surrounding areas, including the Jordan Marsh department store in the city's downtown area and the Boston Young Men's Christian Union. An early etching completed shortly after the hospital was opened shows the slight differences between Nathaniel Bradlee's architectural drawings submitted in 1876 and the asylum as it stood on completion in 1878. The sketch shows couples walking arm in arm along the drive and up the hospital's stately walkways. (Left, John Gray; below, Danvers Archival Center, Danvers, Massachusetts.)

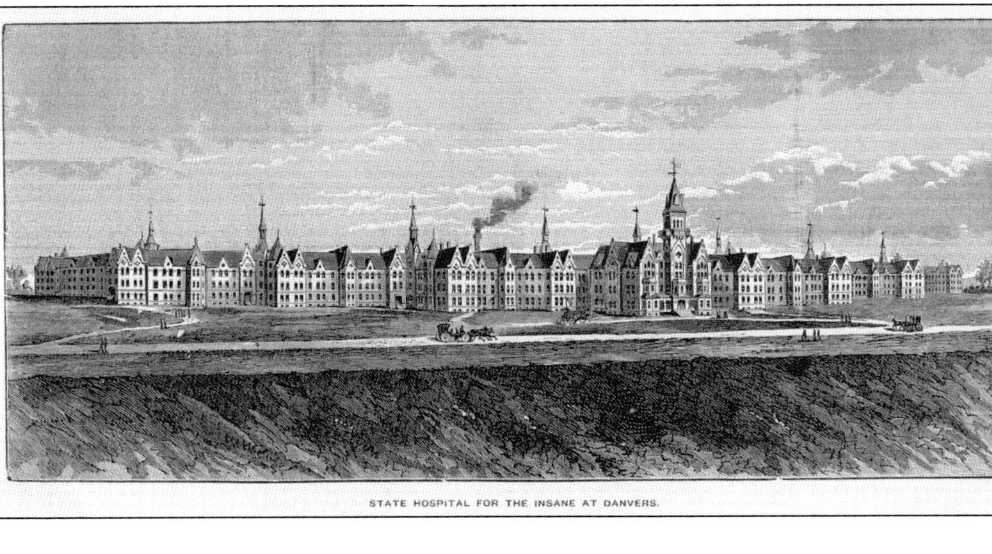

STATE HOSPITAL FOR THE INSANE AT DANVERS.

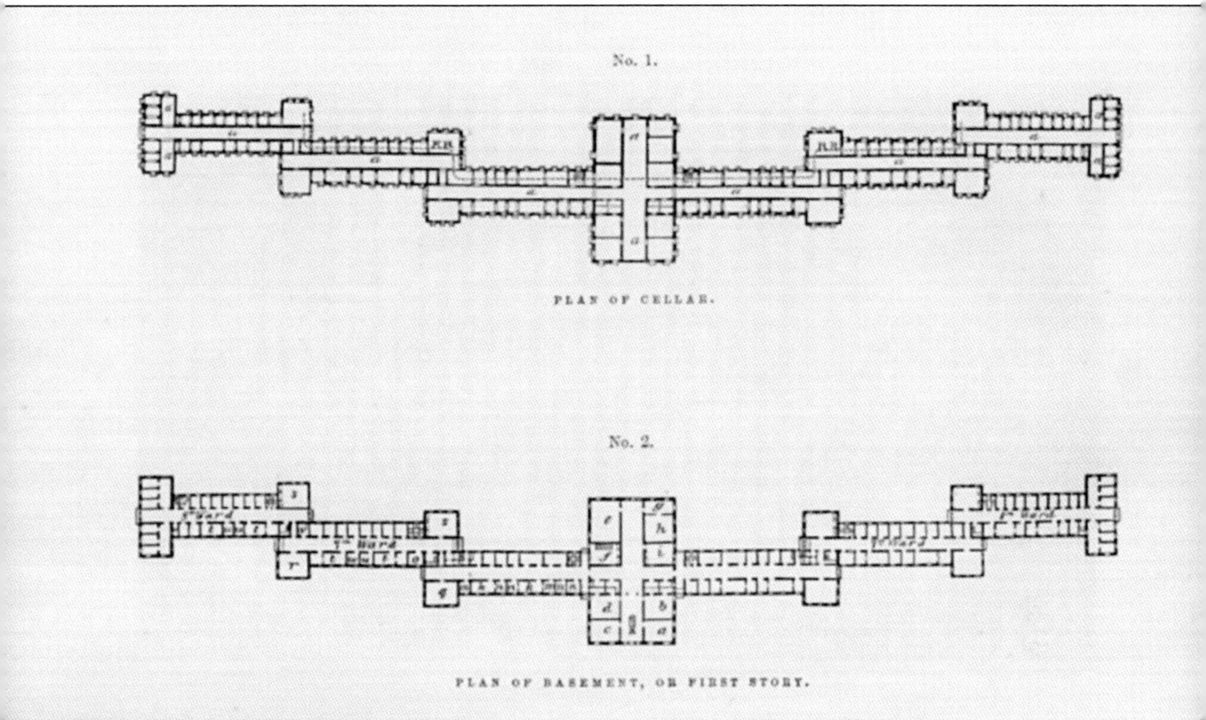

Dr. Thomas Story Kirkbride, a founder of the American Psychiatric Association, was the chief proponent of the centralized plan, a single building to serve the entire patient population that was built upon in all 30 states in existence at the time. The finished hospital floor plan measured an astonishing 313,000 square feet and was 1,100 feet in length. The three-and-a-half-story Kirkbride Complex was designed for a total of 258 patients housed in six separate wings, while the attic infirmaries could house 30 additional patients. Two extra wings for excited patients were connected to the main building at right angles by octagonal entrance towers. (John Gray.)

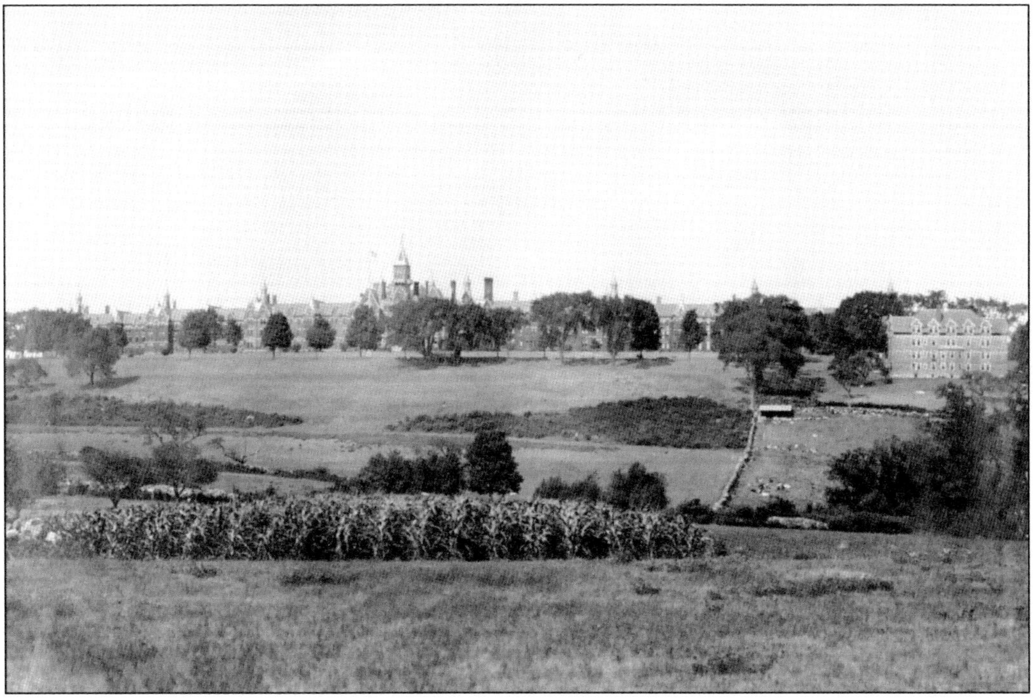

Early on, there were a number of complaints about cost overruns incurred during construction of the asylum. Additional appropriations were requested before construction even began, as the plans for the hospital did not allow for unexpected expenses that were mounting quickly. The architect's estimates were not accurate and it was suggested that costs could have been reduced by choosing a "less steep site." In spite of the numerous infusions of money, the final construction was still found wanting. After a number of rainstorms, it was discovered that the outer walls of the hospital needed pointing and painting as a great deal of water damage had been found inside. Ceilings and plaster walls were stained, water seeping in through badly laid brickwork. (Above, Massachusetts Archives; below, Danvers Archival Center, Danvers, Massachusetts.)

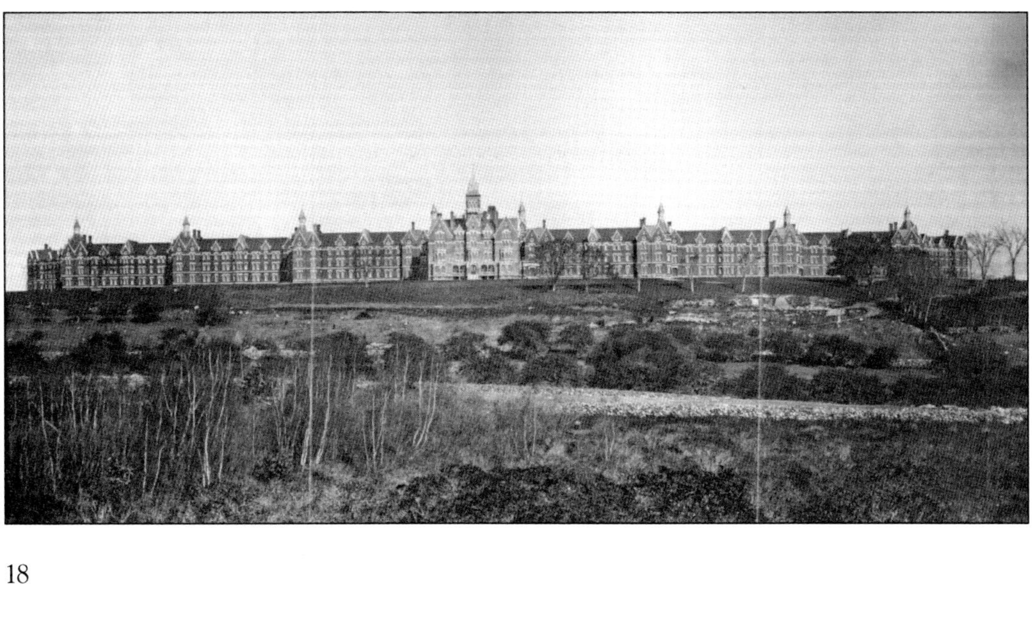

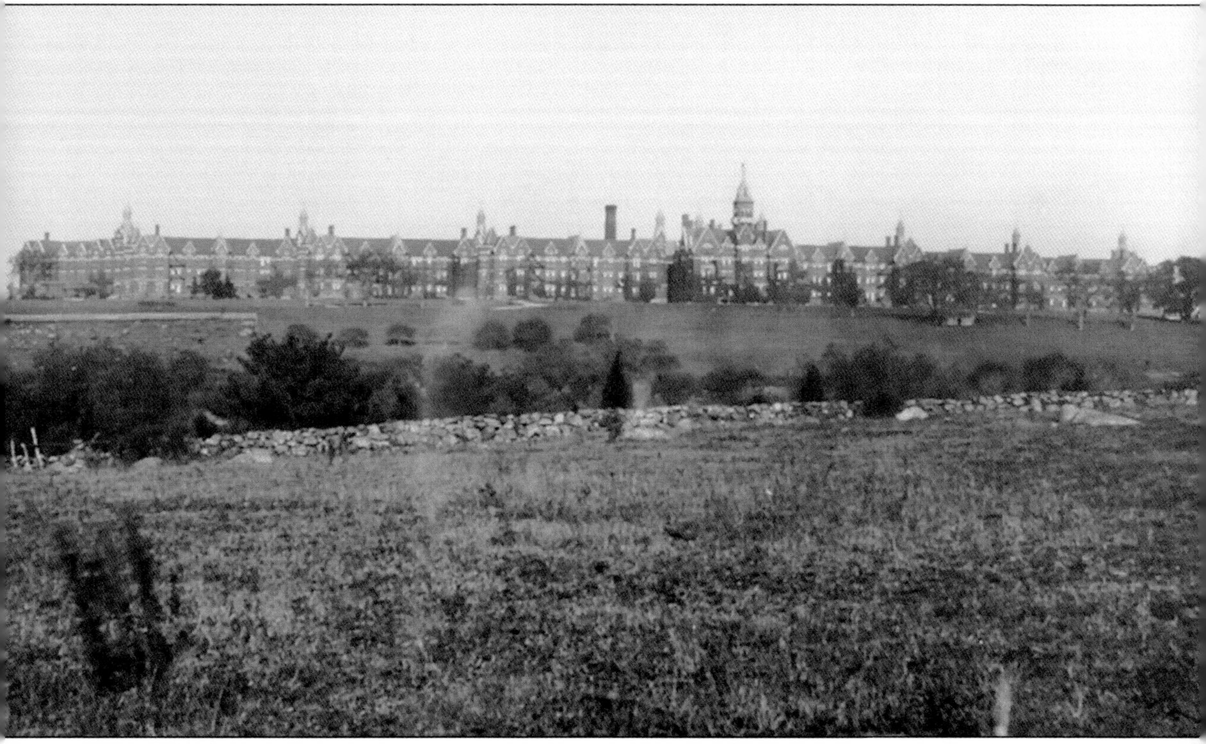

Clement Walker, medical advisor to the State Lunatic Hospital Danvers, wrote in 1875, "A hospital structure—plain and simple but complete in all of its appointments—shall crown Hathorne Hill, with its wealth of pure water and purer air and its broad landscapes of beauty stretching out on every side." This excerpt is from the *Report of the Progress Made by the Commissioners in the Erection of a State Hospital for the Insane at Danvers.* (Danvers Archival Center, Danvers, Massachusetts.)

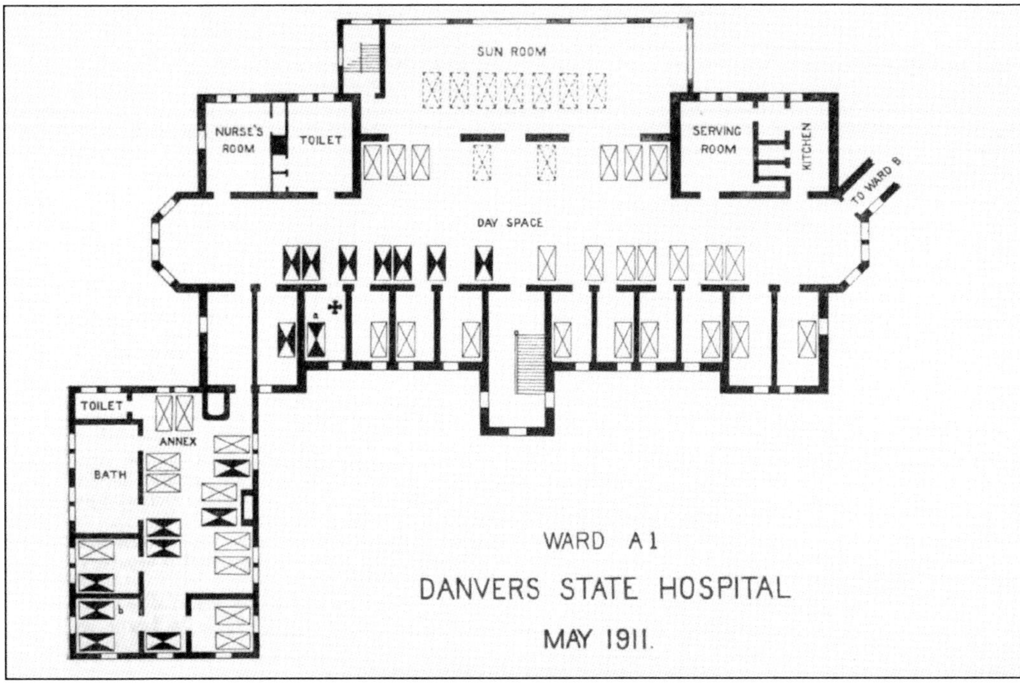

This architectural drawing from 1911 shows the basic layout of one of the wards. Each ward had its own sunroom, communal day room, and kitchen. In the early part of the 20th century, before the patient census exceeded the hospital's capacity, each patient had his or her own private room with a view of the grounds at the back of the hospital and a shared bath. Below is an image of a congregate patient room, likely in the annex of one of the wards. (Above, John Gray; below, Danvers Archival Center, Danvers, Massachusetts.)

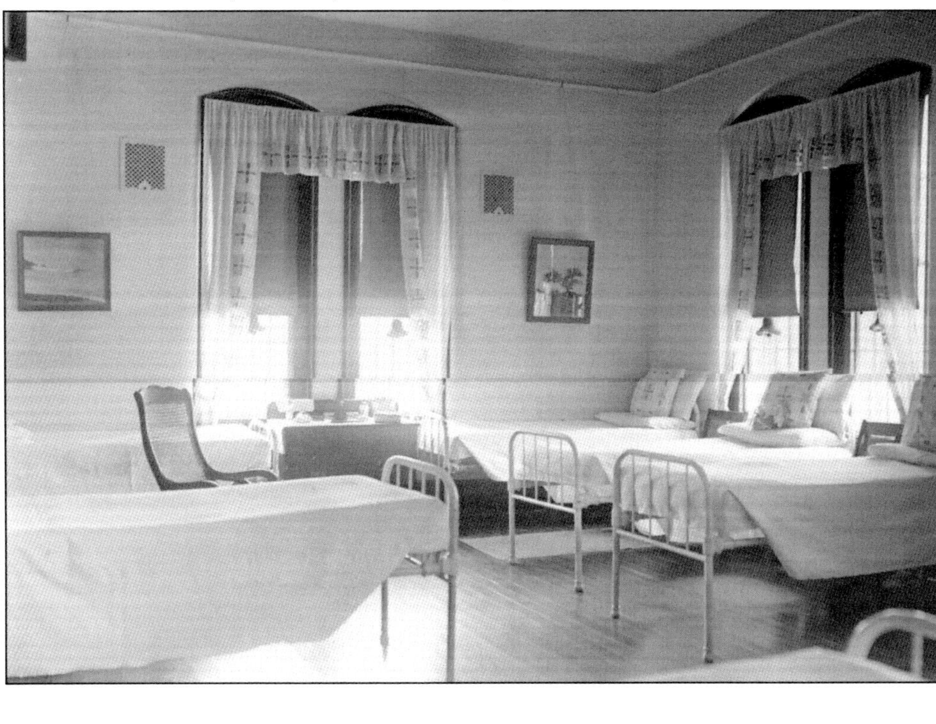

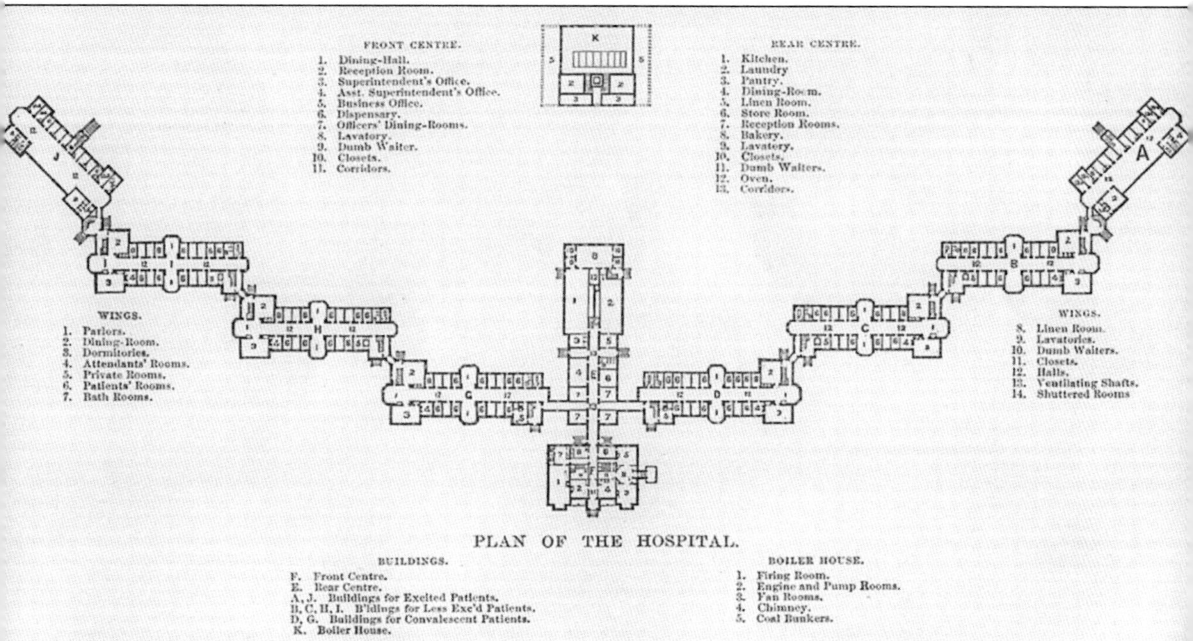

Each Kirkbride hospital built in the United States was constructed on the same basic floor plan, which looked from the air like a bat with its wings outstretched, the wards stepped back from the center, yet each individual hospital boasted at least one unique feature that was a mark of that hospital's particular architect. As can be seen from the annotated floor plan, the wing tips of the ward halls were extended by the addition of towers that joined the excited wards with the buildings for "less excited" patients. Each ward had its own parlor and dining room with shared bathrooms, while the main administration building at the heart of the bat wing housed the superintendent's office, the assistant superintendent's office, the dispensary, and the business office. (John Gray.)

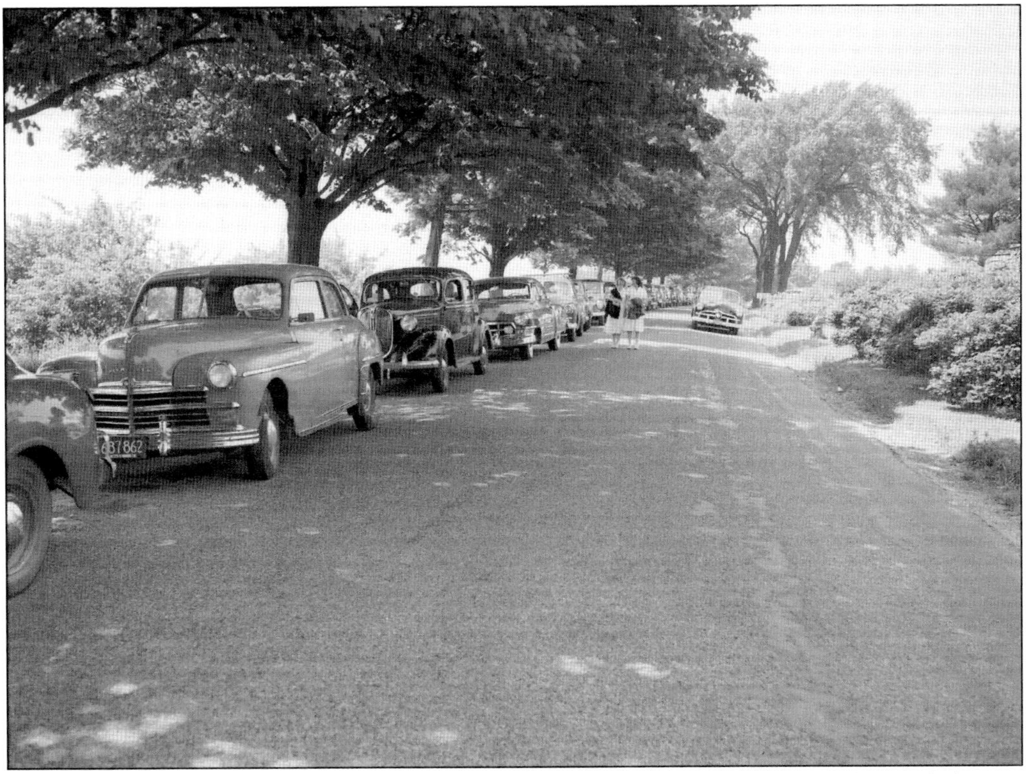

The elegant drive up to the Kirkbride was lined with flowering lilac bushes and provided views of Putnam and Peabody from the peak of its 197-acre campus. The drive crested in front of the eight-foot double oak doors with etched-glass windows that opened into the main administration offices. Sharon Cook, a now retired occupational therapist, recalls doing her internship at Danvers. Though the Kirkbride was already closed, she often walked up the hill to see the old buildings. After the hospital's official closure, Sharon was able to transplant one of the lilac trees from the main drive before they were removed. (Both, David Walsh.)

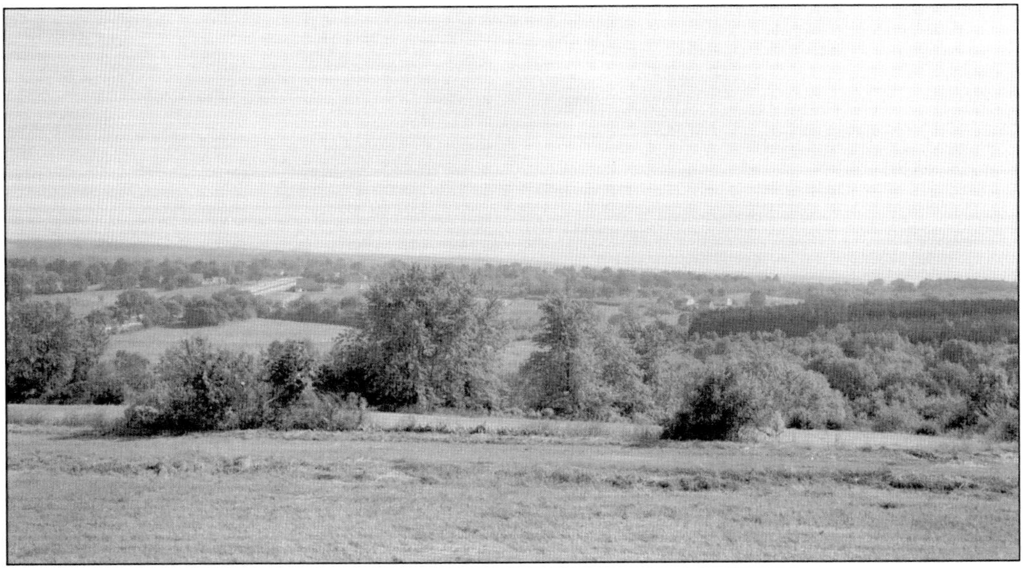

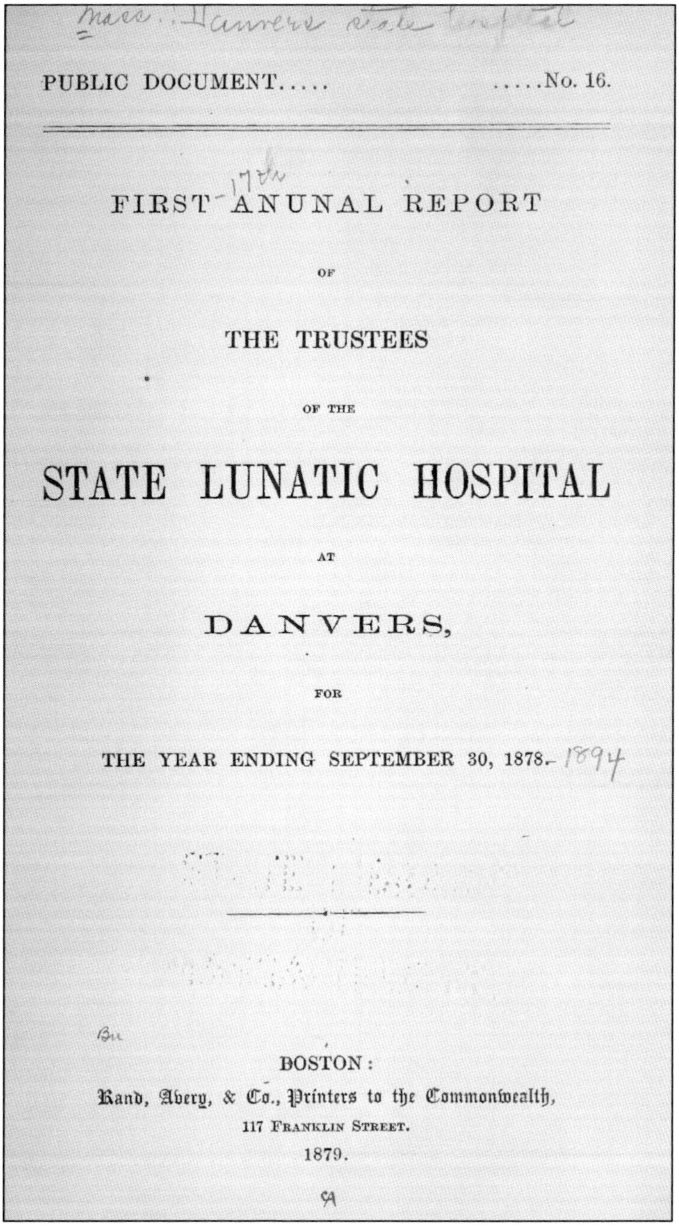

PUBLIC DOCUMENT..... .....No. 16.

FIRST ANUNAL REPORT

OF

THE TRUSTEES

OF THE

STATE LUNATIC HOSPITAL

AT

DANVERS,

FOR

THE YEAR ENDING SEPTEMBER 30, 1878.

BOSTON:

Rand, Avery, & Co., Printers to the Commonwealth,

117 Franklin Street.

1879.

The Trustees of the State Lunatic Hospital at Danvers submitted their first annual report at the close of 1878 after receiving control of the hospital from the state commissioners. Dr. Calvin S. May was appointed first superintendent of Danvers State Insane Asylum. May previously served as the assistant physician at the Connecticut Hospital for the Insane, then went on to serve at Danvers until 1880. In the first year, 305 patients were admitted; 71 of whom were discharged soon after, making the average population throughout the year approximately 114. The clinical study of the causes of insanity and mental infirmity began almost immediately with an eye to becoming a hospital that might cure as many patients as possible, rather than immediately becoming a custodial asylum for the chronic insane. The trustees intended to provide the greatest comfort and attention possible in an institution for the insane, hoping to rank among the most "useful of the charitable institutions of the Commonwealth." (John Gray.)

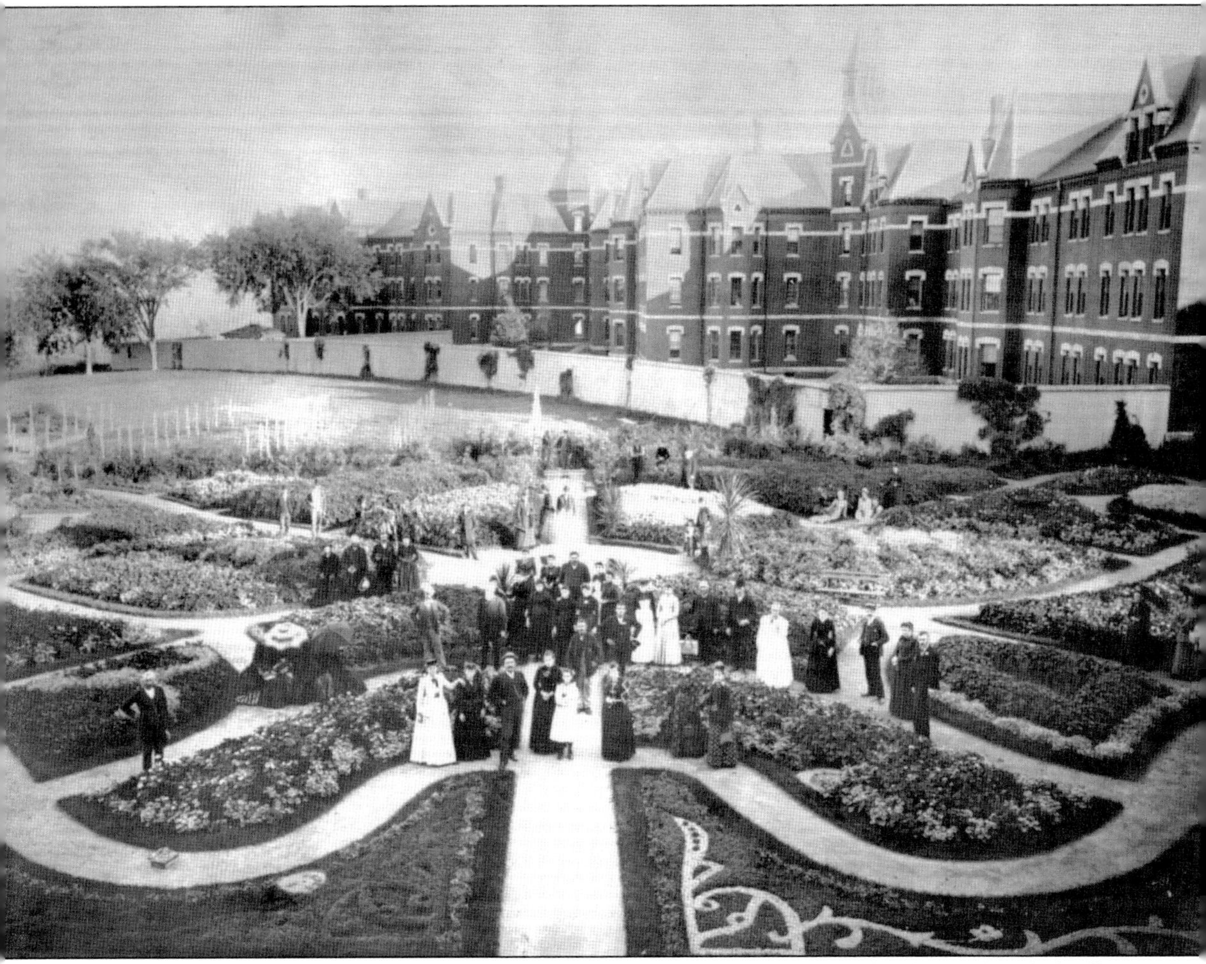

The Danvers State Insane Asylum officially opened on May 1, 1878, after being handed off to the first board of trustees in 1877. The hospital received its first patients on May 13 and official notice of the hospital's opening was provided to the public. The influx of patients was gradual but steady, and the trustees too were proud that Calvin May was upholding their vision of the hospital being curative. They lauded May's ability to manage the hospital while remaining attentive to the patients and making them as comfortable as possible, no matter how short their stay. (John Gray.)

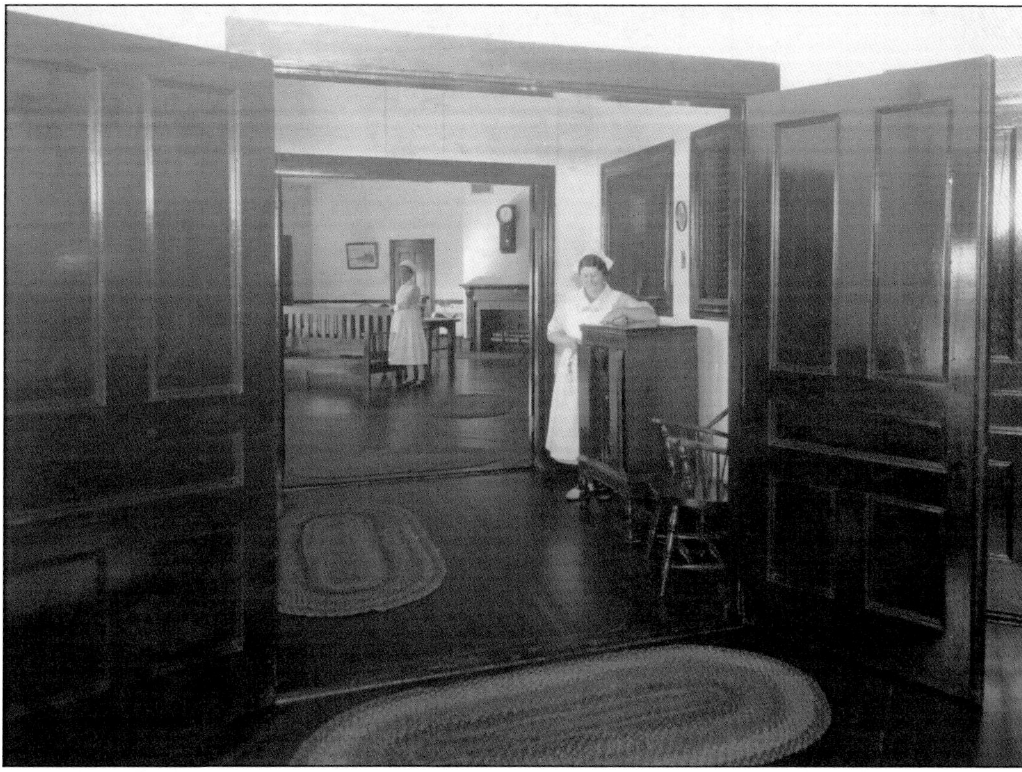

Though there were no exact specifications for the interior of the hospital, it followed the most modern thinking of the time. The walls were plastered in light colors with curved surfaces that extended to doorways and entryways. Floors were bare hardwood, and in some cases the ceilings were made of decorative tin. In its first year of operation, the asylum was only partially filled and the furnishings incomplete. However, the trustees noted that a very modest budget was followed when procuring stylish and "modern" furniture and finishes for all areas of the hospital. (Both, Danvers Archival Center, Danvers, Massachusetts.)

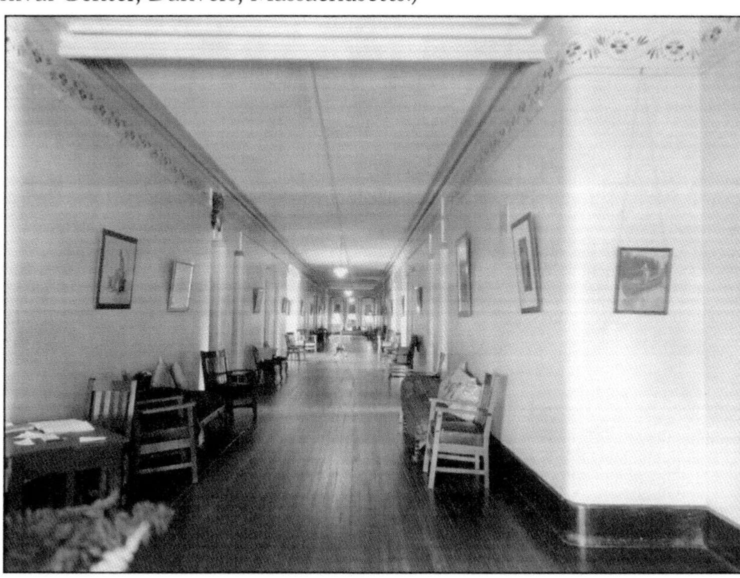

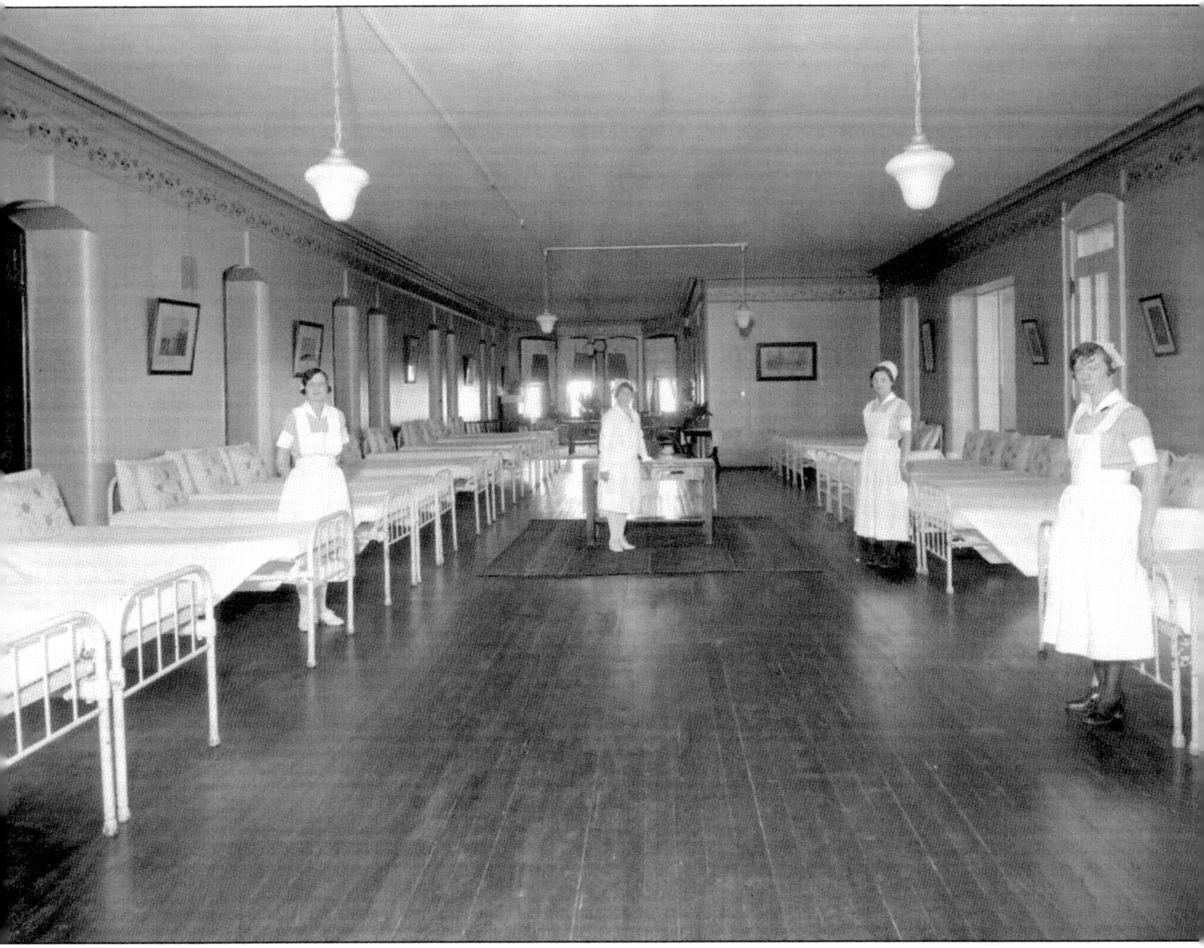

According to an article titled "Opening of the Hospital" in the May 18, 1878, edition of the *Danvers Mirror*, the decor and splendor of the new institution were meant to aid in destigmatizing the institutional environment. The article goes on to refer to the hospital's exquisite surroundings, the buildings a "veritable nest of beauty." Often, the townspeople would pack picnic lunches and visit the campus on open Sundays, just to come and view the architecture. An 1889 article in the *New York Mail* said of the grounds, "Probably nowhere in New England . . . are there more wonderful floral designs." (Danvers Archival Center, Danvers, Massachusetts.)

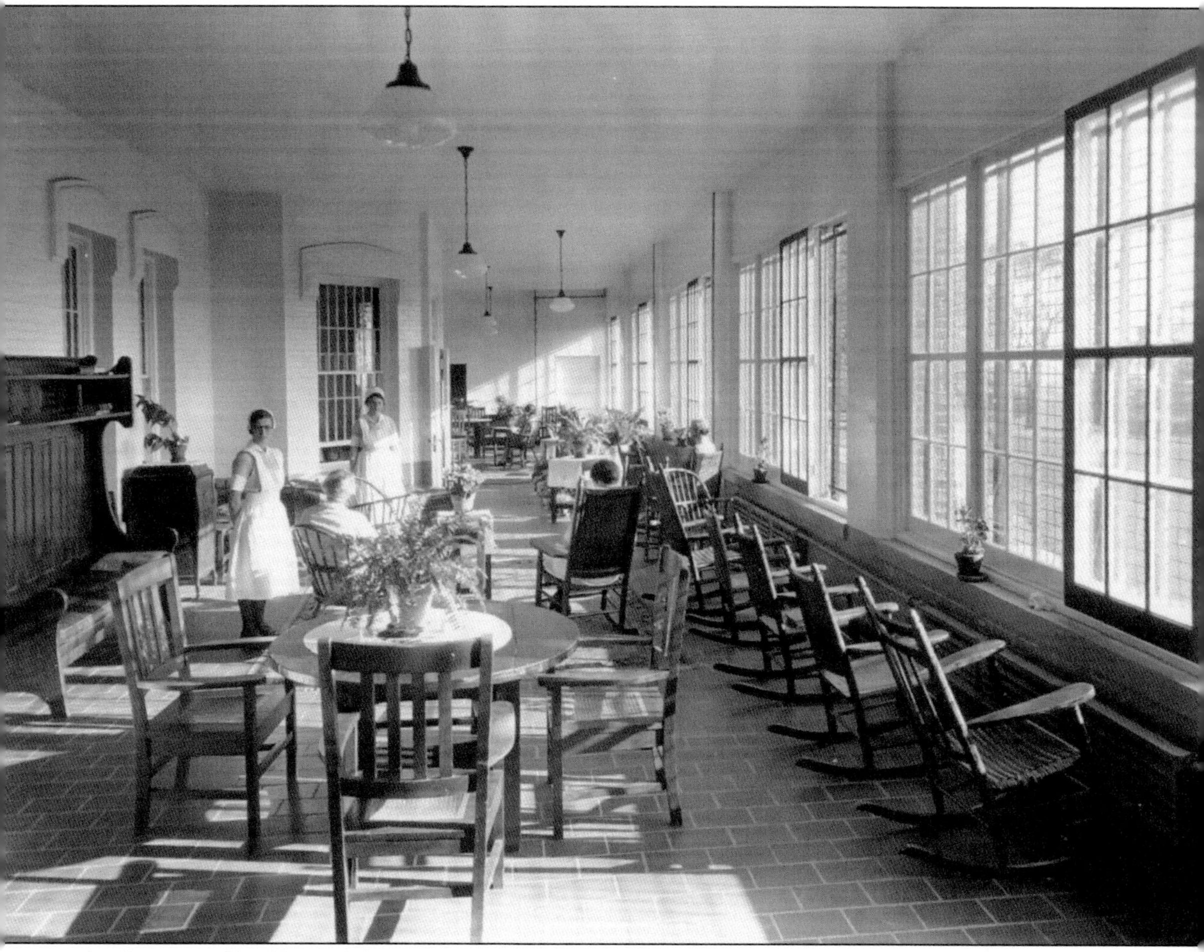

The design and building of the state hospital at Danvers sparked bitter controversy, raising concerns that the grandeur of the building was overshadowing its true purpose. After numerous requests for more funding, many were concerned that the Danvers Insane Asylum was already exceeding its intrinsic worth, taking money away from already open and operating asylums. Even Pliny Earle, superintendent of Northampton State Hospital, "decried the trend to excessive ornamentation in hospital architecture . . . suggesting that 'domes, towers and turrets are very appropriately situated . . . at universities . . . but are scarcely appropriate when they stand as monuments over the misfortunes and the miseries of men.'" (Danvers Archival Center, Danvers, Massachusetts.)

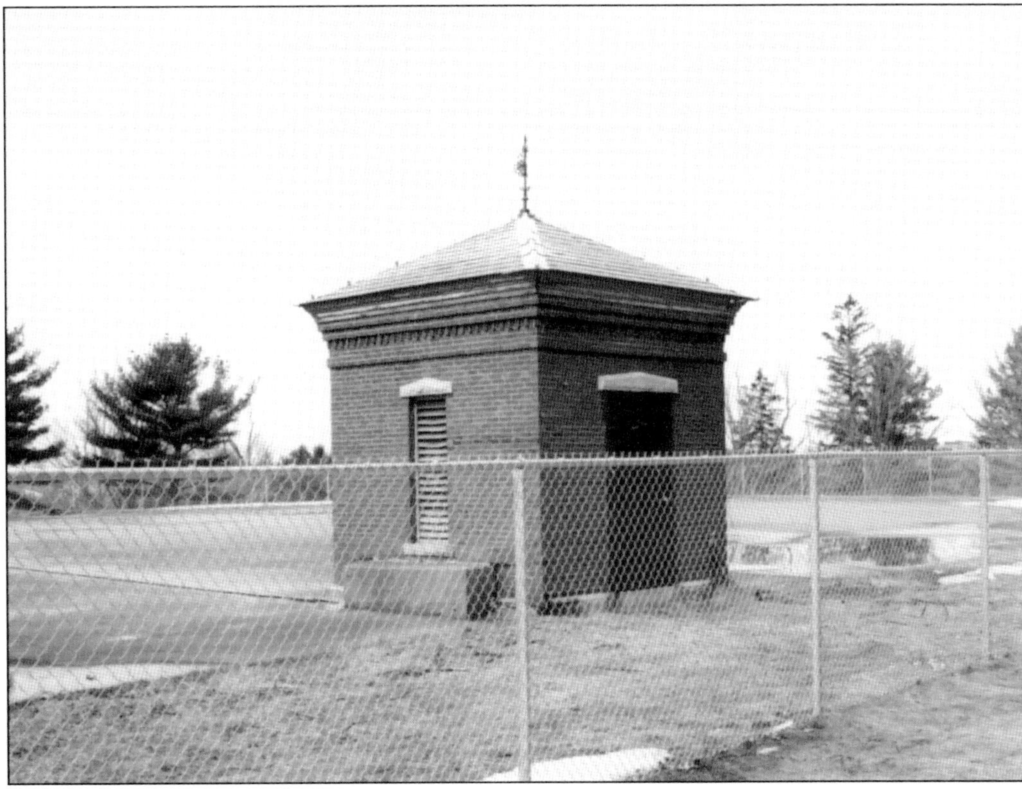

A major part of mental health "therapy" at the time was the provision of fresh, clean water. The town offered its own water supply from Middleton Pond, and in 1876, the town agreed to build a waterworks at a cost of $12,500 plus $1,000 each year for 20 years from the state. An intermediate reservoir would be built on the grounds to supply a gravity fed system that would fill ten 5,000-gallon tanks in the hospital's attic. (Danvers Archival Center, Danvers, Massachusetts.)

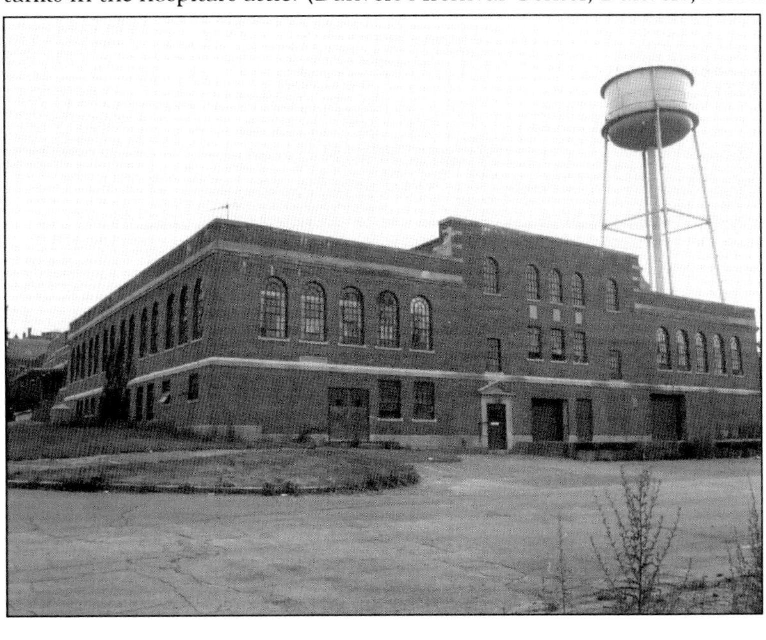

The powerhouse at Danvers State Hospital was built at the height of the Industrial Revolution and was meant to generate power for the 700,000-square-foot Kirkbride. It would later be enlarged, and three more boilers were added to provide adequate steam heat and power for the institution. (John Gray.)

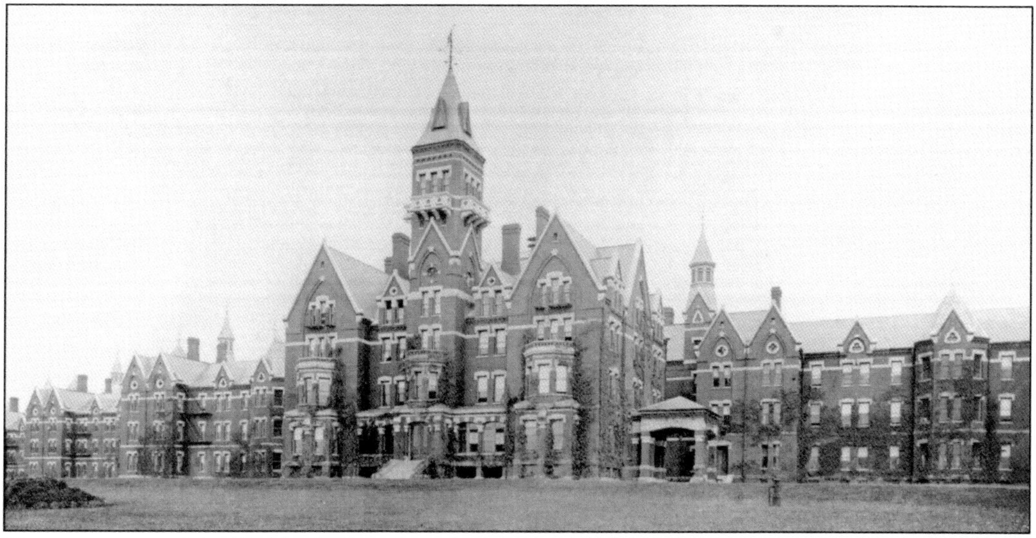

The main core of the Kirkbride, known as Front Centre, housed the administrative offices with a service area directly behind. Rear Centre housed the hospital's bakery, kitchen, and laundry with dining and reception rooms for the attendants. A chapel occupied the second and third floors plus servant bedrooms and storage. (Danvers Archival Center, Danvers, Massachusetts.)

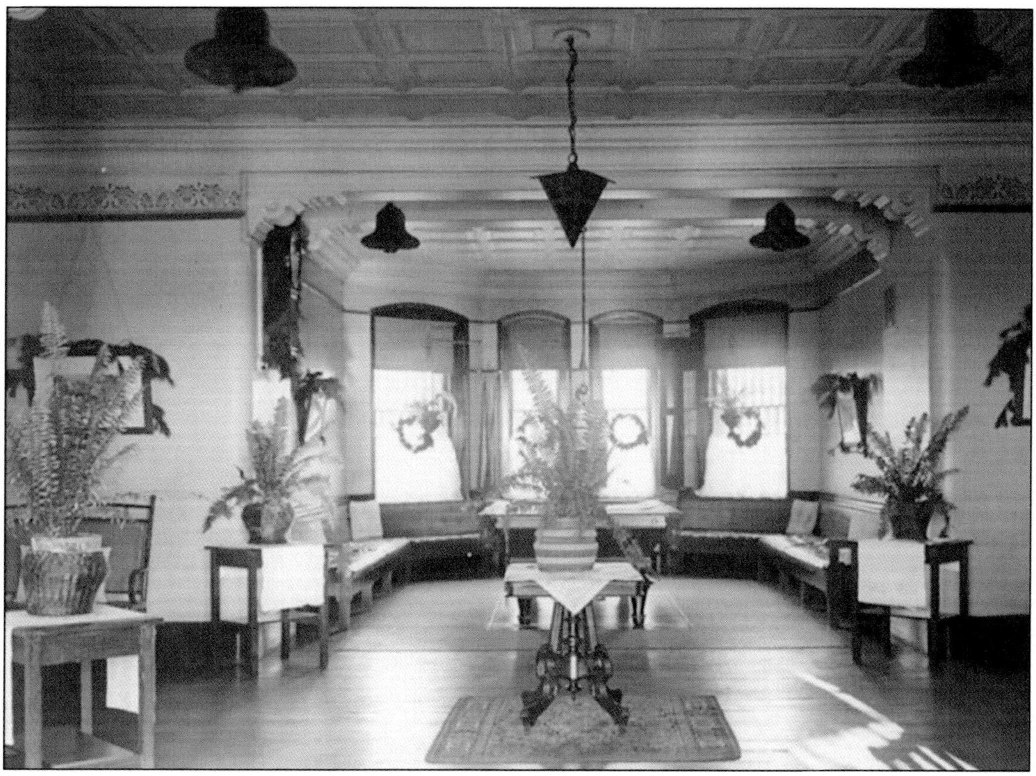

To the left of the main entrance were a number of dining and reception rooms, bathrooms, a pantry, and closets. The superintendent's private and public rooms were to the right along with the apothecary. The floors above were mainly sitting rooms reserved for administrators' families. (Danvers Archival Center, Danvers, Massachusetts.)

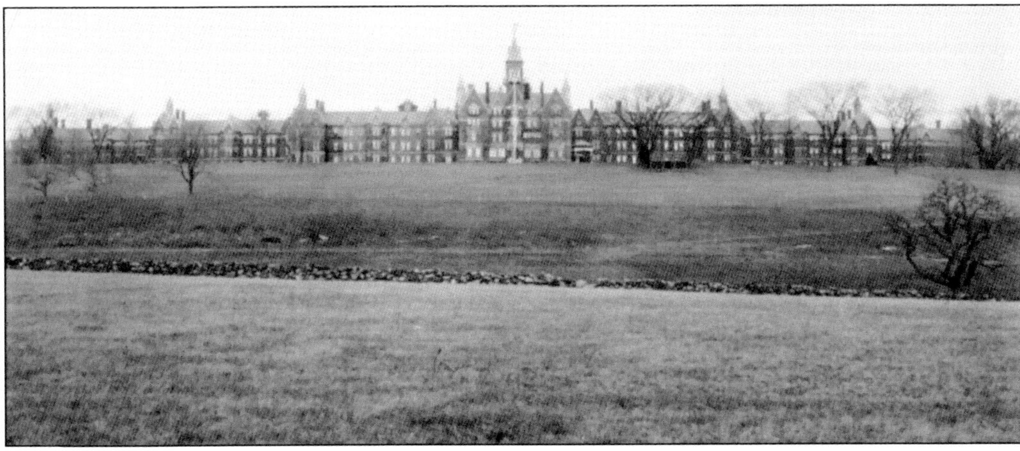

Three stepped-back patient wings stretched from each side of the administration building, with men to the left and women to the right. Each wing, six in total, had its own dining and reception rooms, working fireplaces, and attendants' quarters. Two extra wings, A and J, were connected at a 45-degree angle by octagonal entrance towers and held 72 patients. (Danvers Archival Center, Danvers, Massachusetts.)

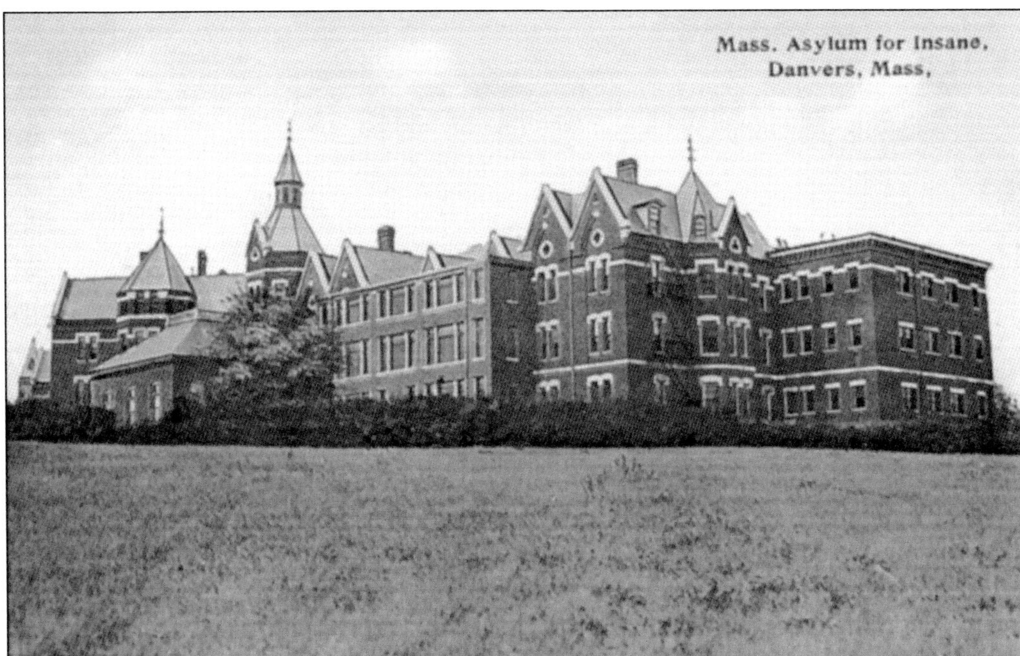

Nearly the entire hospital was constructed of red Danvers brick, manufactured by hand. The length of the building measured 1,180 feet, and one wall alone was nearly a mile long with nearly 240 angles. The windows were wreathed in cut granite, the steps leading to each entrance also made from granite slabs. (John Gray.)

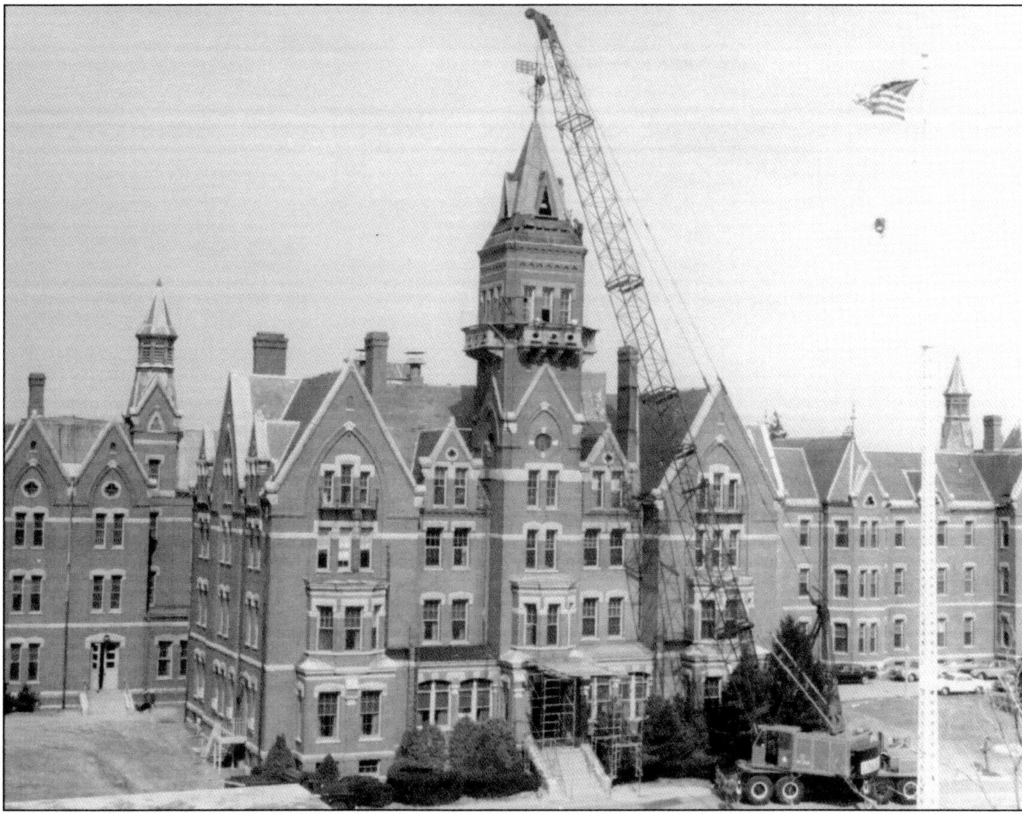

On April 6, 1970, the upper portion of the main administration steeple was deemed unsafe and removed by crane. The tower was too expensive to repair, and it was reported that pieces had begun to fall off. The tower was stored behind the Bonner Building at first but was eventually taken to the dump. For a time, the wrought iron weathervane that graced the tower was stored in the blacksmith shop, but it too was never seen again. AvalonBay recreated the steeple to match the original exactly when building Avalon Danvers. (Above, Danvers Archival Center, Danvers, Massachusetts; below, John Gray.)

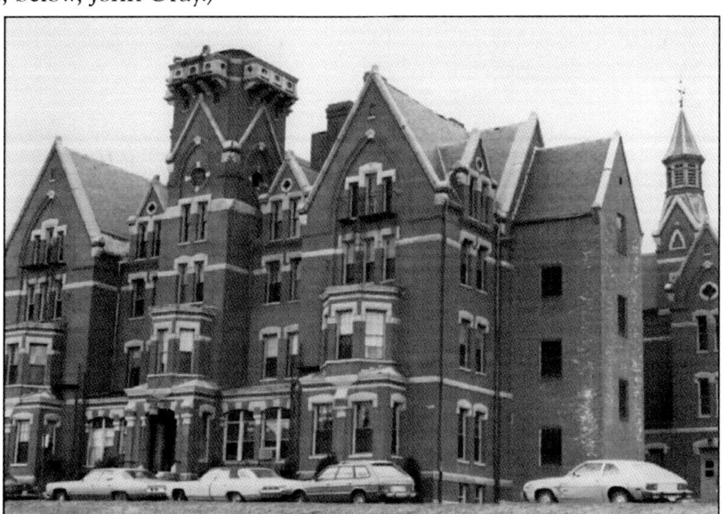

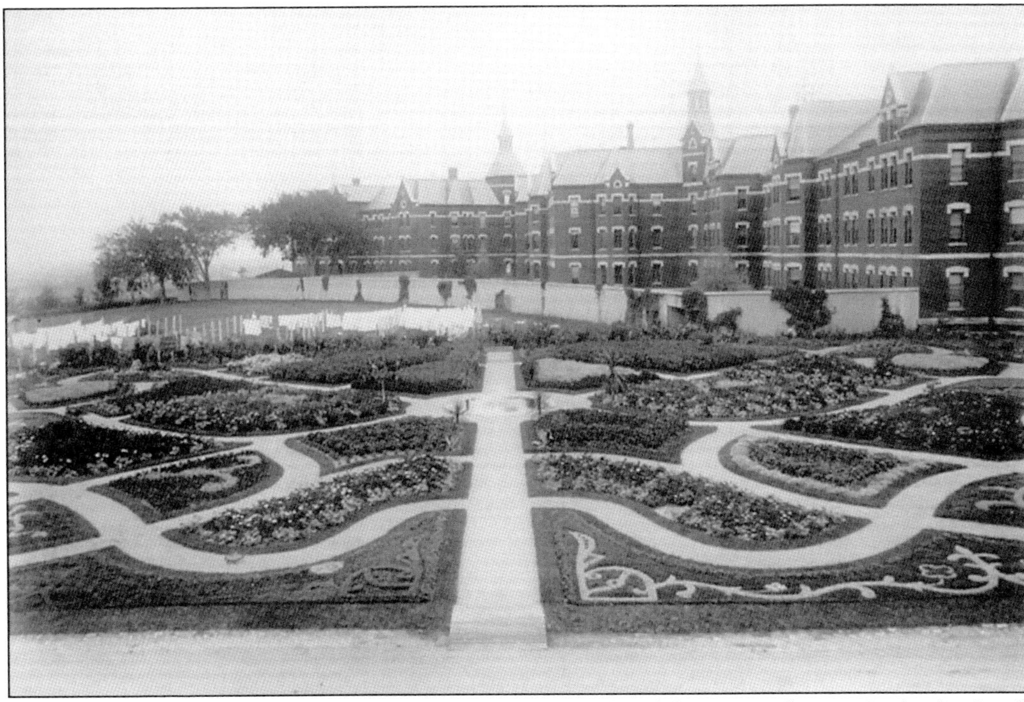

Designed by Italian landscape gardener Ettore Jassinari, the elaborate gardens at the back of each of the male and female wings attracted roughly 12,000 visitors each year. They were comprised of over 100 different beds dotted with grottoes and fountains that fed into pools where more fountains spewed water into the air. Flowers in one bed were laid in the shape of a sundial while another bed formed a calendar in the shape of a scroll. Another was made to announce the weather of the day, while yet another bed marked the four points of a compass. (Both, John Gray.)

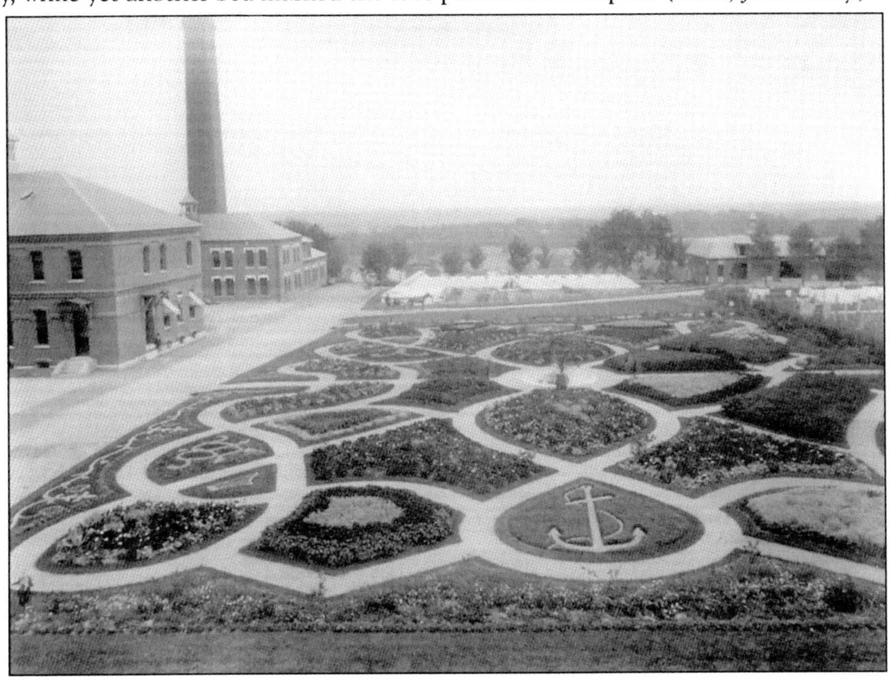

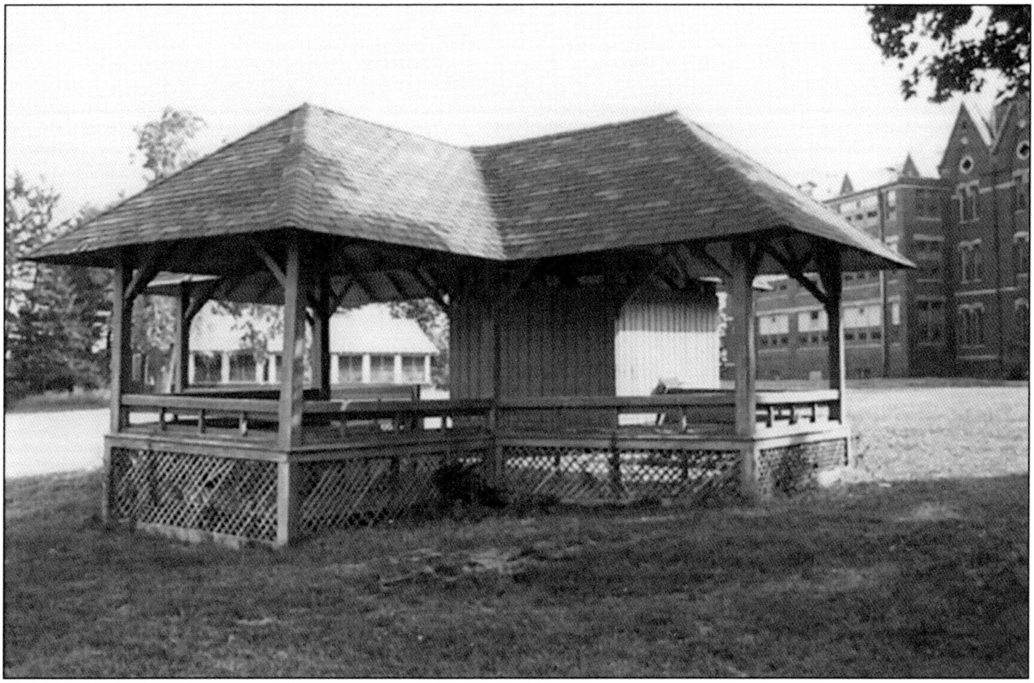

Pavilions, also called summerhouses, were built outside each of the main wings where male and female patients respectively could sit outside and enjoy the air or have a cigarette. The pavilions were also used for picnics and as snack stands during community activities such as the annual country fair. The pavilions, at the back of the hospital, provided a measure of privacy for both patients and staff with views of the farm. Staff occasionally led exercises near the pavilions—presumably so that patients could sit in the shade and rest after participating in activities. (Both, John Gray.)

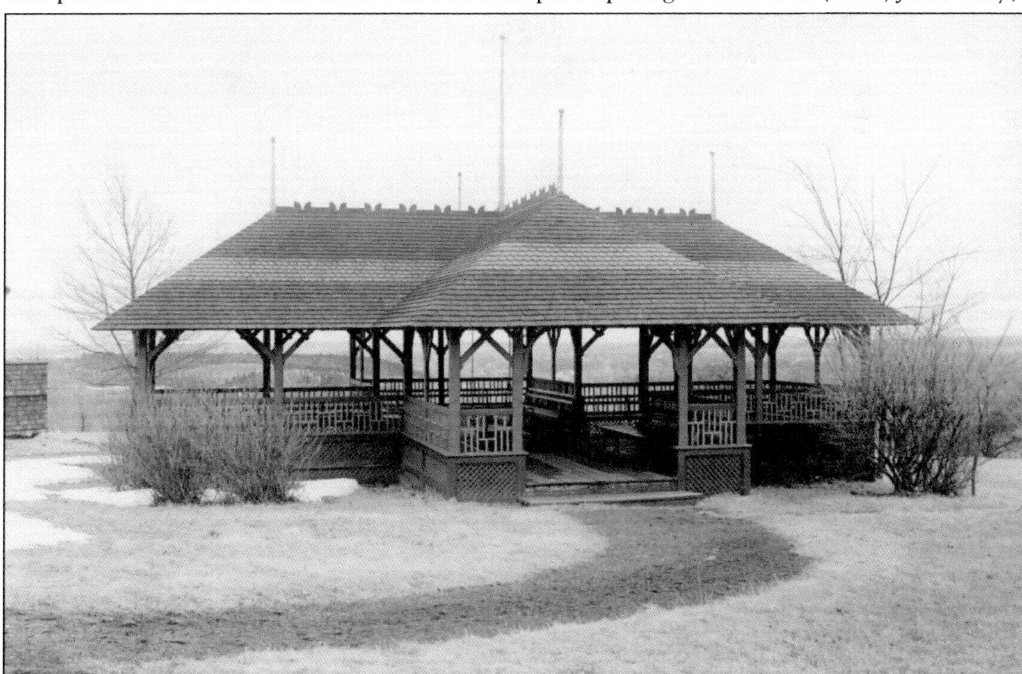

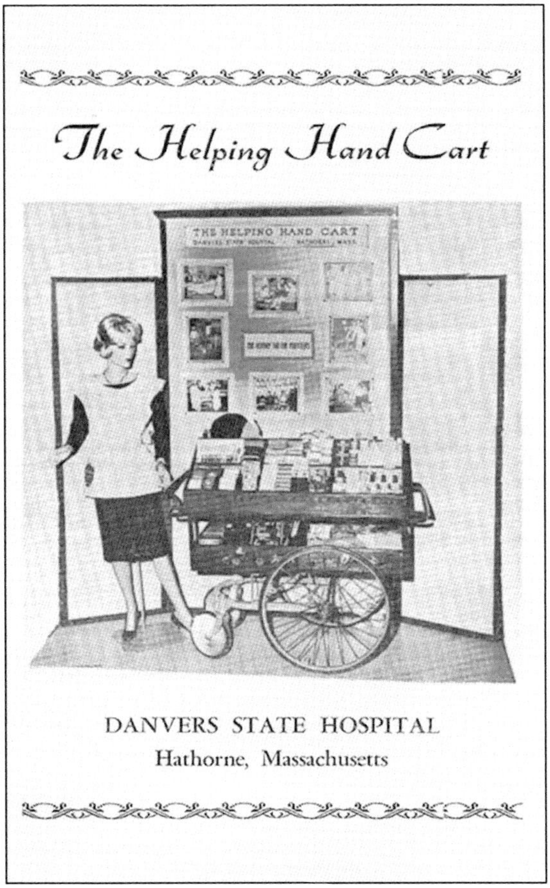

Community presence on the hospital campus was established as early as the 1880s, when visitors would come from the surrounding towns not only to spend time visiting with the patients but also to conduct religious services and lead arts and crafts projects. They also provided patients with small sundries for the "Helping Hand Cart." (John Gray.)

Visitors were welcome at the hospital on any given day. Early postcards such as this one boasted that the campus was easily reached by automobile, railroad, and trolley from the surrounding towns of Salem, Middleton, and Lawrence. Visitors often brought flowers of their own for the patients as well as books and magazines. (David Walsh.)

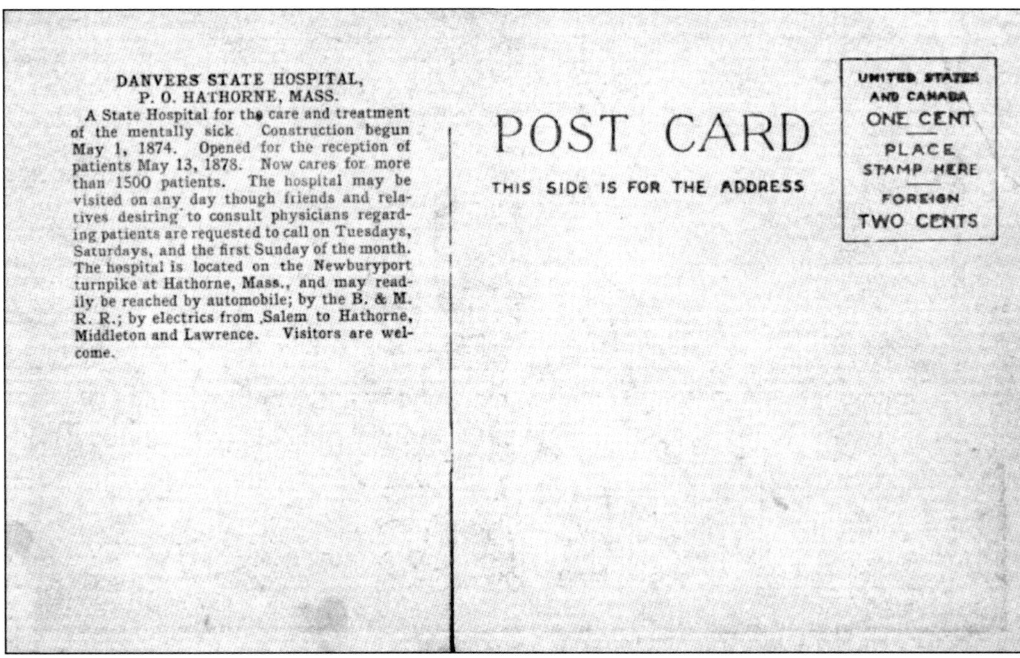

DANVERS STATE HOSPITAL,
P. O. HATHORNE, MASS.

A State Hospital for the care and treatment of the mentally sick Construction begun May 1, 1874. Opened for the reception of patients May 13, 1878. Now cares for more than 1500 patients. The hospital may be visited on any day though friends and relatives desiring to consult physicians regarding patients are requested to call on Tuesdays, Saturdays, and the first Sunday of the month. The hospital is located on the Newburyport turnpike at Hathorne, Mass., and may readily be reached by automobile; by the B. & M. R. R.; by electrics from Salem to Hathorne, Middleton and Lawrence. Visitors are welcome.

POST CARD

THIS SIDE IS FOR THE ADDRESS

UNITED STATES AND CANADA ONE CENT
PLACE STAMP HERE
FOREIGN TWO CENTS

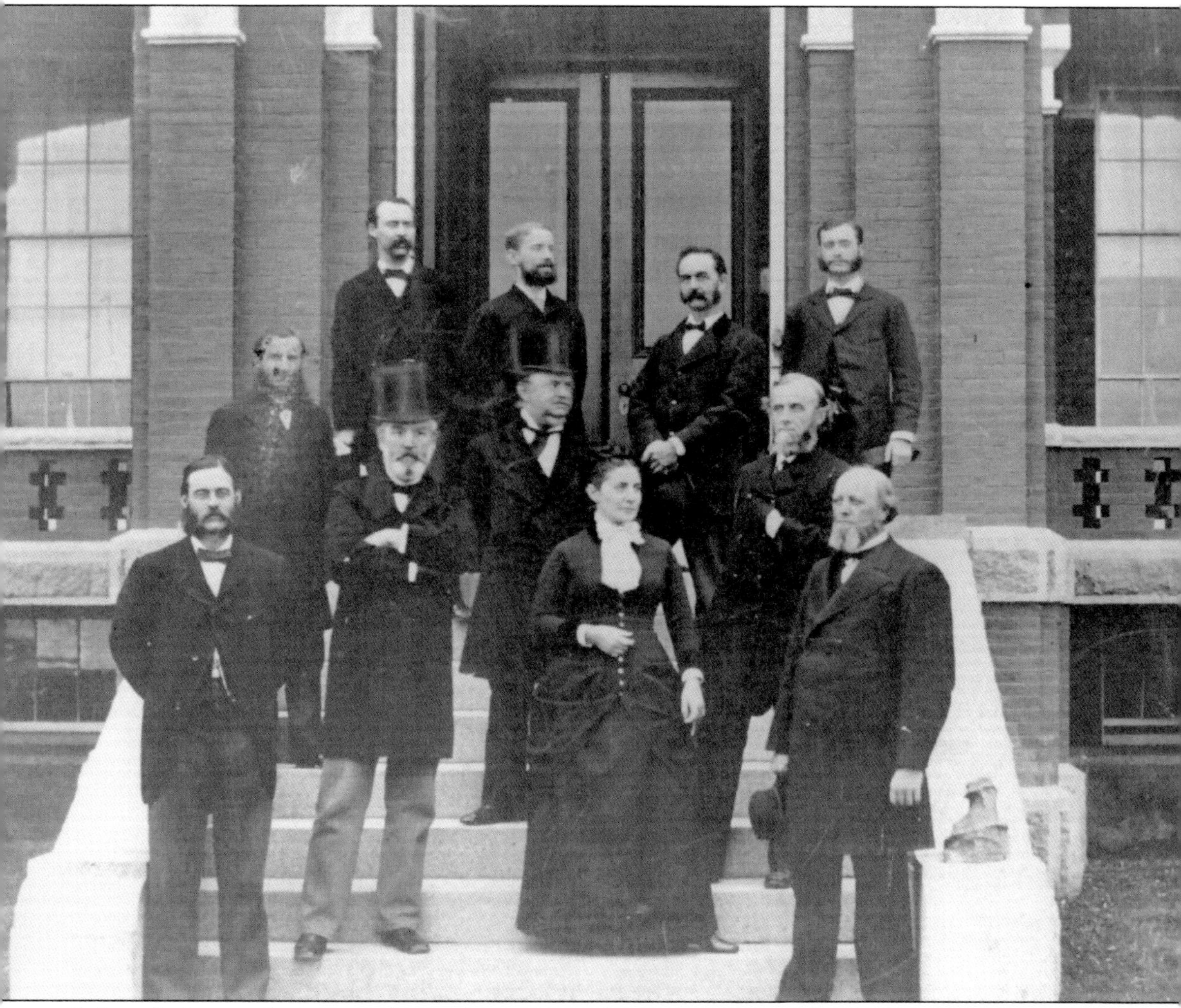

Before the hospital was turned over the trustees, the Commissioners for the Erection of a State Asylum in Danvers issued their own report in 1876. Construction was underway but, as noted in the report, the original allocation of funds would not be nearly enough to carry out the architect's vision. The site had to be graded as Hathorne Hill had an extreme elevation unsuitable for building as it stood. A water supply would also need to be secured in order to keep the building of the asylum on schedule and have a drainage system built. Ultimately, with expenses mounting, the Massachusetts State Legislature approved another $600,000 on top of the initial sum of $900,000 already allocated for the asylum in hopes that the hospital would be ready to open its doors in spring of 1878. (Danvers Archival Center, Danvers, Massachusetts.)

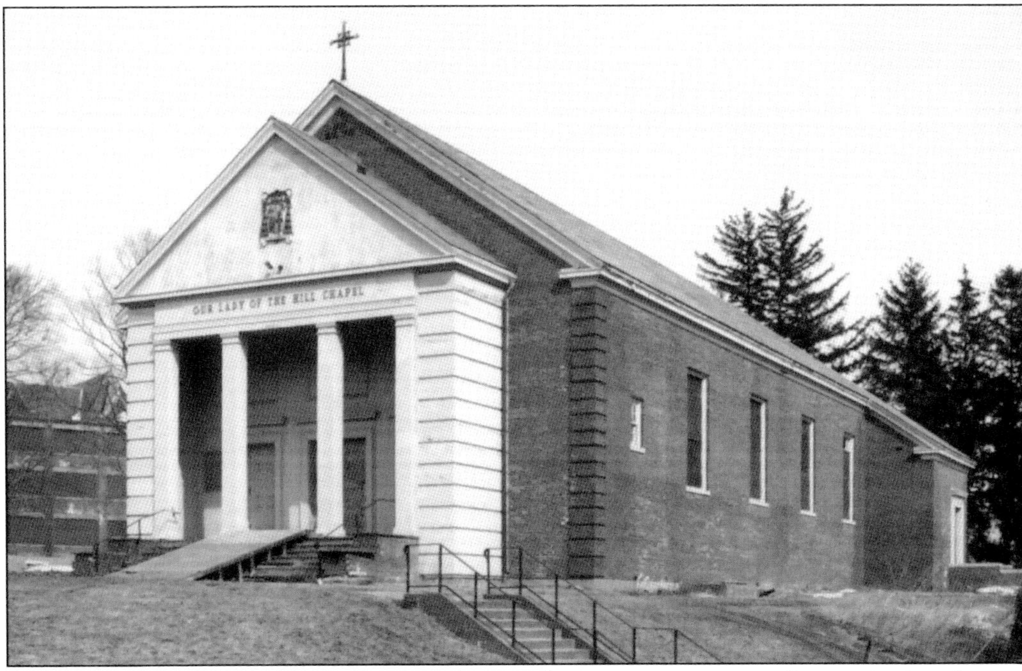

The chapel, which served both the attendants and patients, was originally attached to the rear of the main Kirkbride building, along with the kitchens, laundries, and staff dormitories. After many years, the trustees' requests for an expansion were heard, and a larger, free standing chapel was built on the grounds. In 1955, Our Lady of the Hill Chapel opened for services. A second chapel, St. Luke's, was added in 1964 to serve the Protestant population of staff and patients at Danvers. Both remained in operation until the early 1990s. (Above, Danvers Archival Center, Danvers, Massachusetts; below, John Gray.)

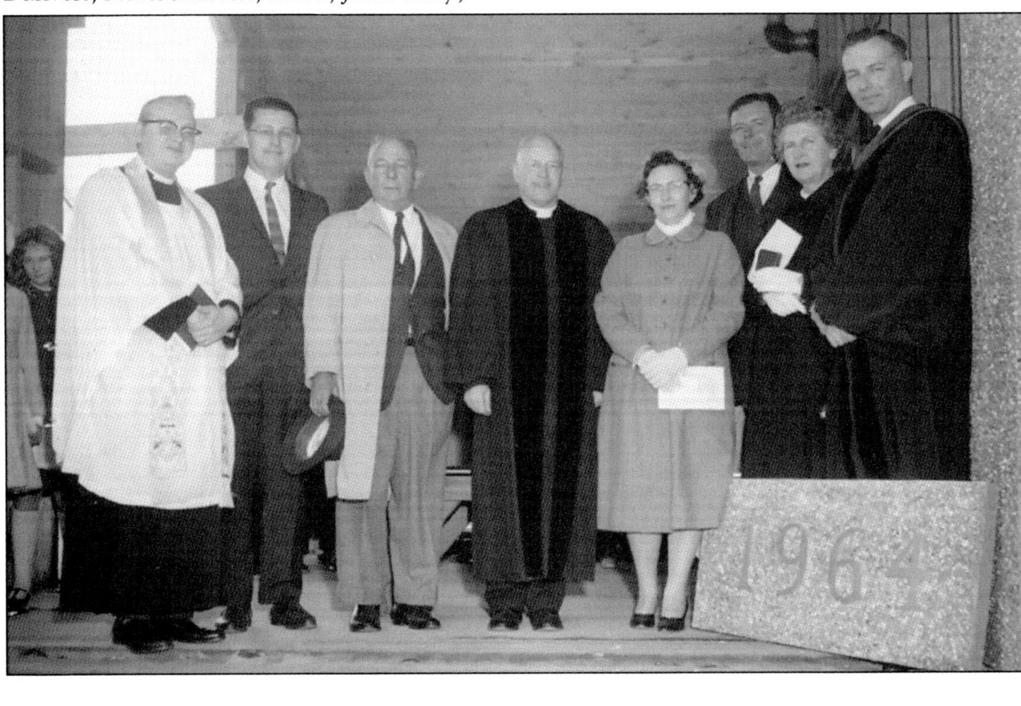

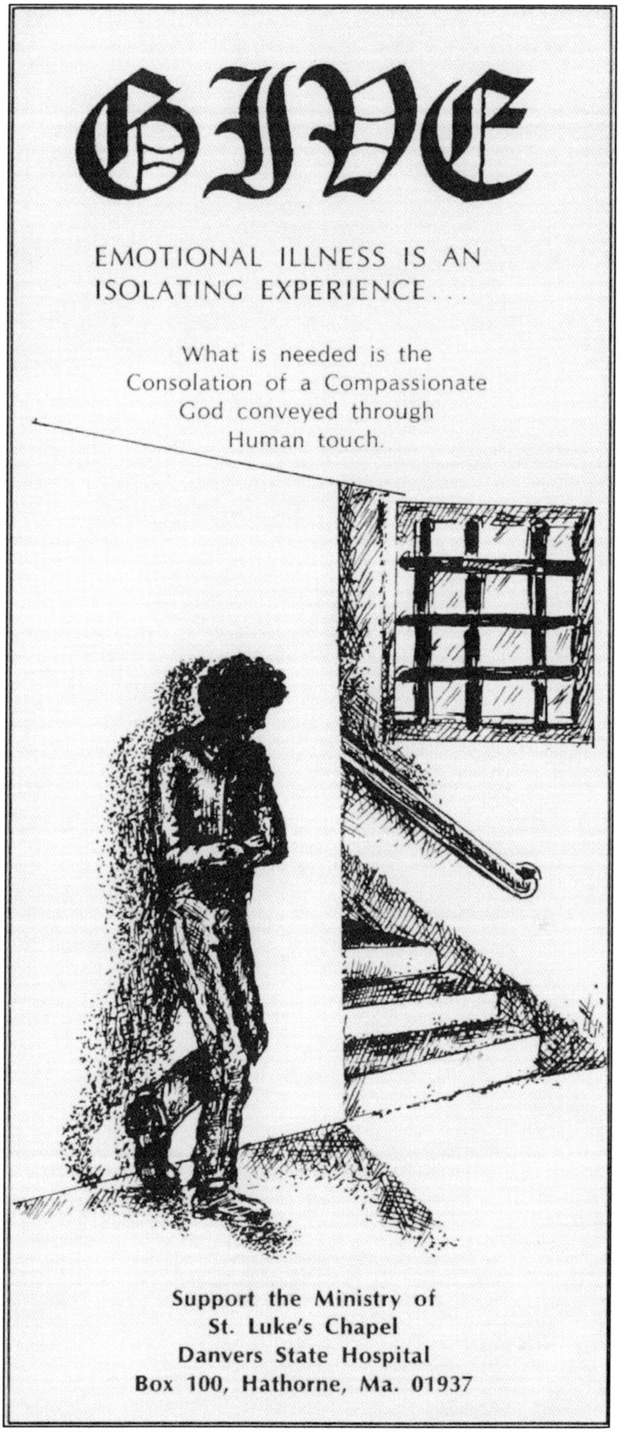
GIVE
EMOTIONAL ILLNESS IS AN
ISOLATING EXPERIENCE . . .
What is needed is the
Consolation of a Compassionate
God conveyed through
Human touch.
Support the Ministry of
St. Luke's Chapel
Danvers State Hospital
Box 100, Hathorne, Ma. 01937

The ministry of St. Luke's chapel was dedicated to community outreach in an effort to connect the patients at Danvers State Hospital to the outside world. Recognizing the complicated nature of mental illness, this St. Luke's pamphlet implores the community to donate to the chapel ministries. (Amanda Kohut.)

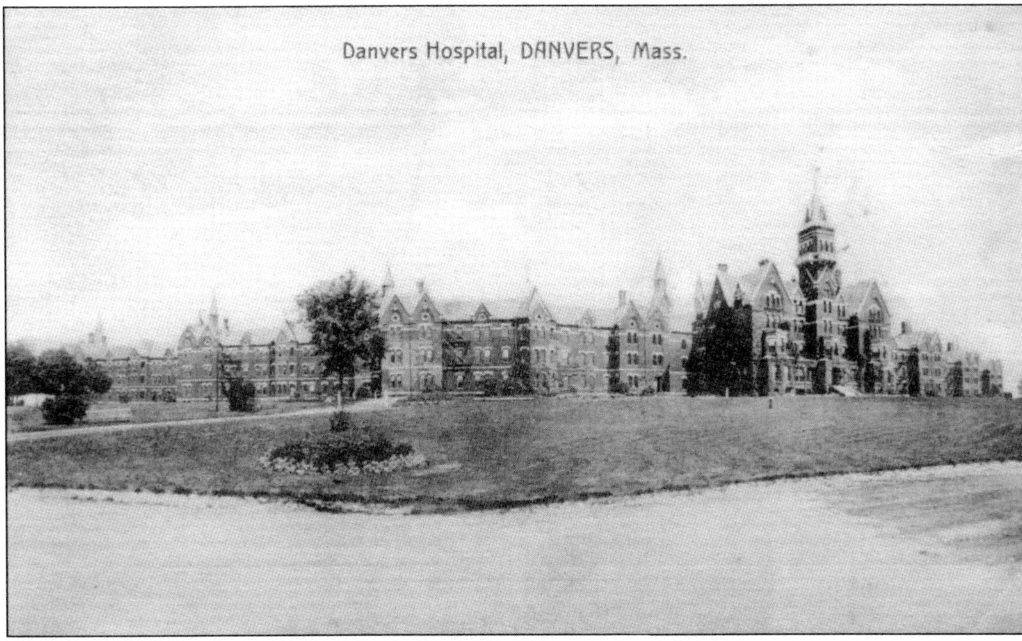

This early postcard of Danvers shows the main administration building of the Kirkbride flanked by the wards with the female wing to the left and the male wing to the right. The front lawn slopes down Hathorne Hill to the ridge overlooking the town. (Danvers Archival Center, Danvers, Massachusetts.)

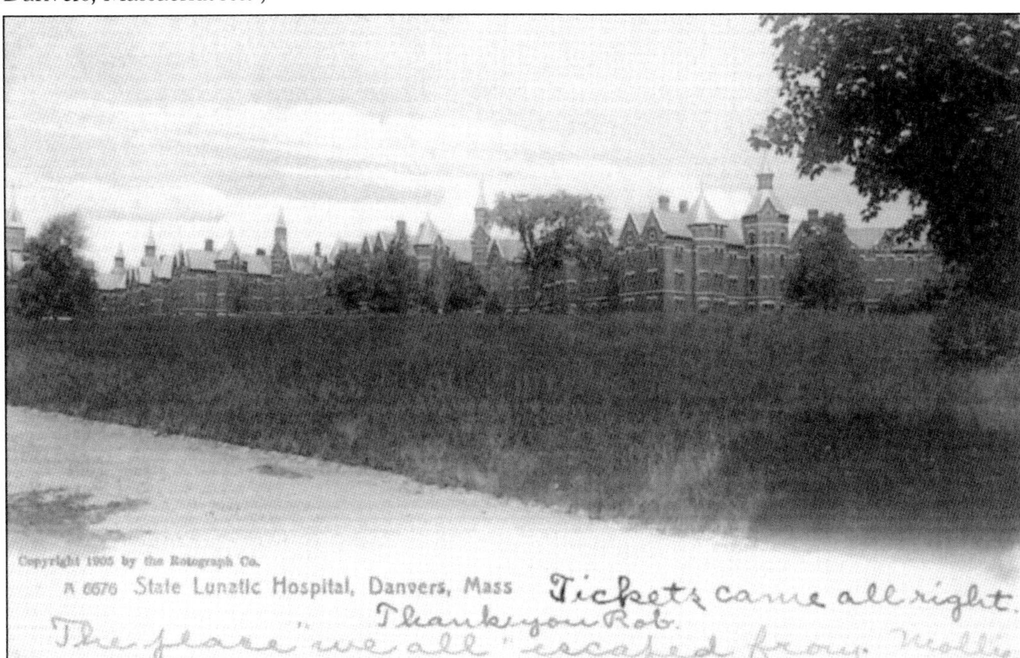
Copyright 1905 by the Rotograph Co.
A 6676 State Lunatic Hospital, Danvers, Mass
Tickets came all right.
Thank you Rob.
The place "we all" escaped from. Mollie

A second vintage postcard, dated July 4, 1906, shows the Danvers Asylum photographed from the base of Hathorne Hill, where the railroad tracks ran. In three short years, the name of the institution would change from Danvers Insane Hospital to Danvers State Hospital—its second renaming. (John Gray.)

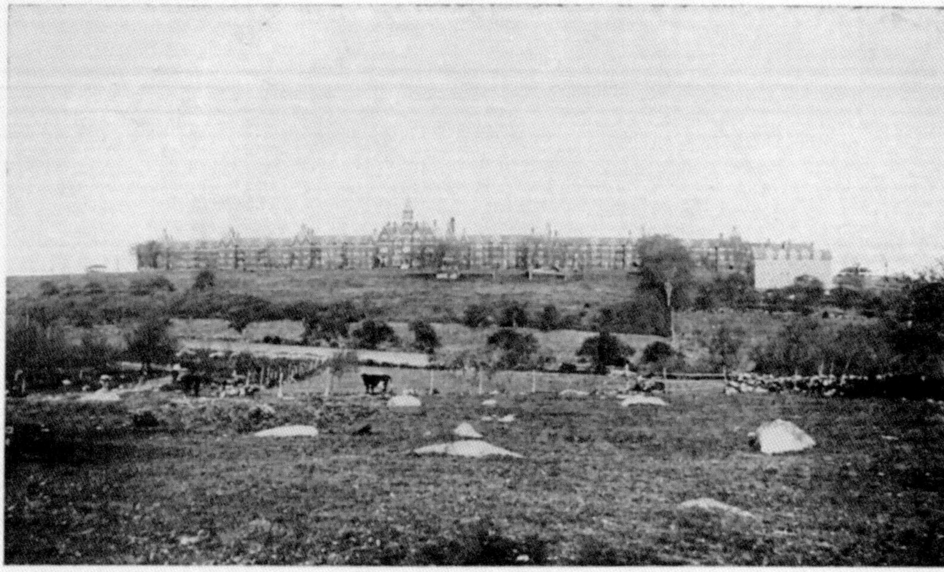

DANVERS STATE HOSPITAL

Most of the hospital's food was grown on site, the asylum farmlands being expansive. As early as the mid-1880s, the farm boasted an annual profit of nearly $30,000. It became the site of a progressive method called "contour farming," in which crops were planted in curved rows that aided in soil conservation. (Both, John Gray.)

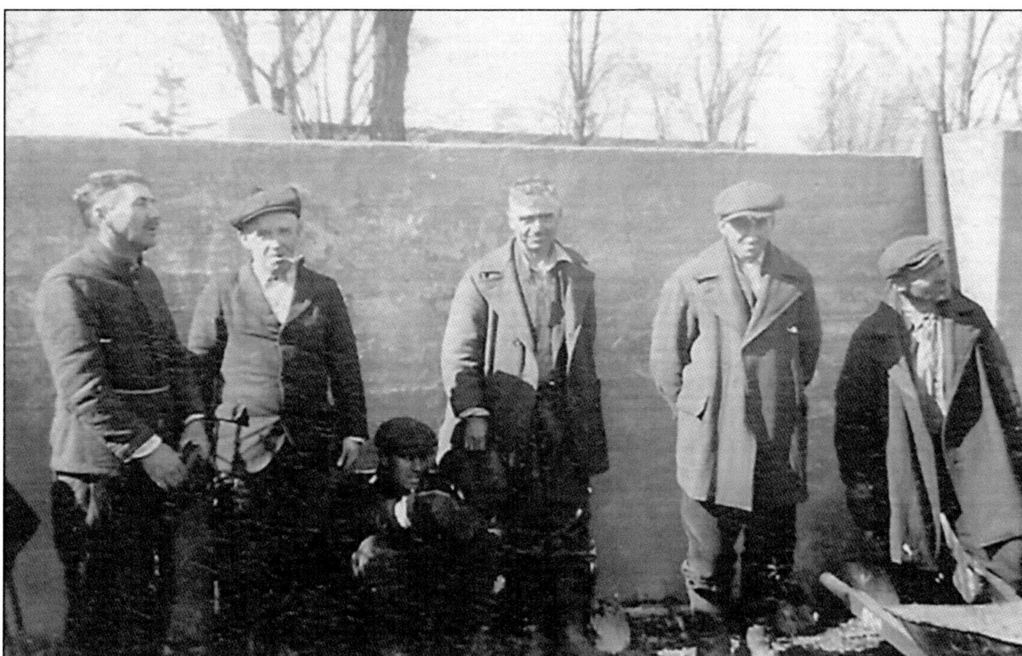

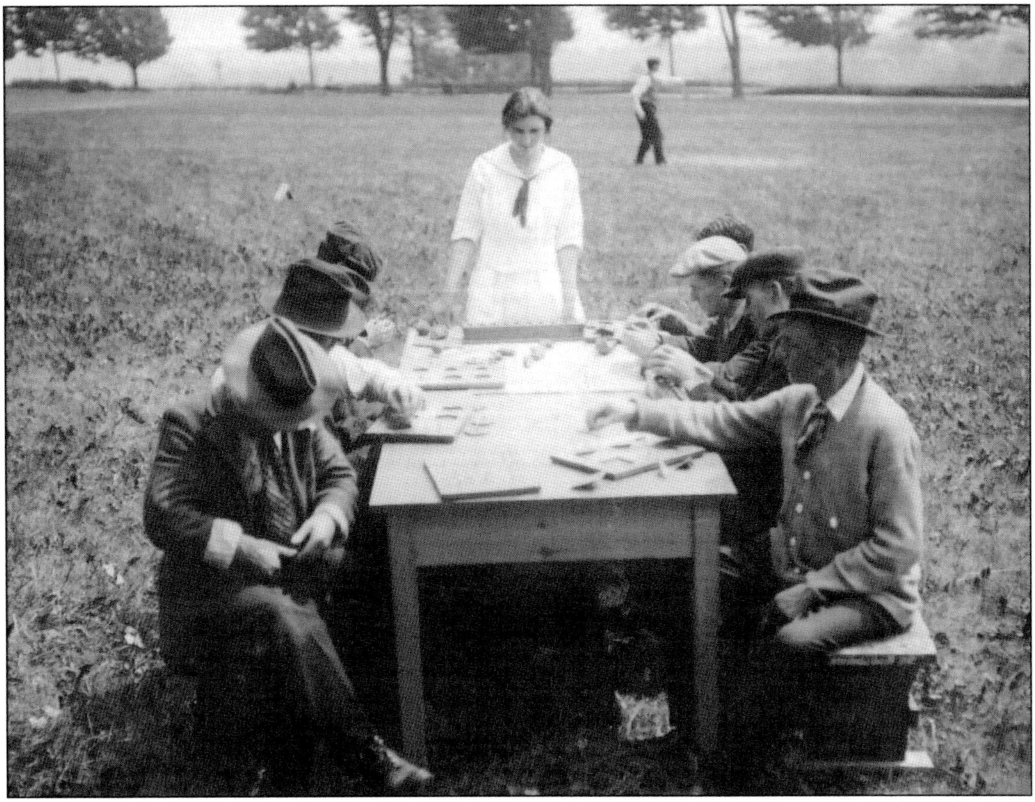

Though Danvers is now considered infamous for its history of mistreatment and deplorable conditions, the asylum was once considered a model of humanistic care dedicated to avoiding both seclusion and restraints to amend behaviors. The staff believed that mechanical restraints and seclusion should remain a last resort for only the most complicated of cases. Instead, patients were afforded exercise, fresh air, and in some cases, freedom to walk the grounds. A major tenet of moral treatment was fresh air and exercise, an integral part of a patient's treatment, which might include gardening, working on the farm, or participating in organized outdoor events. (Both, Ben Kenny.)

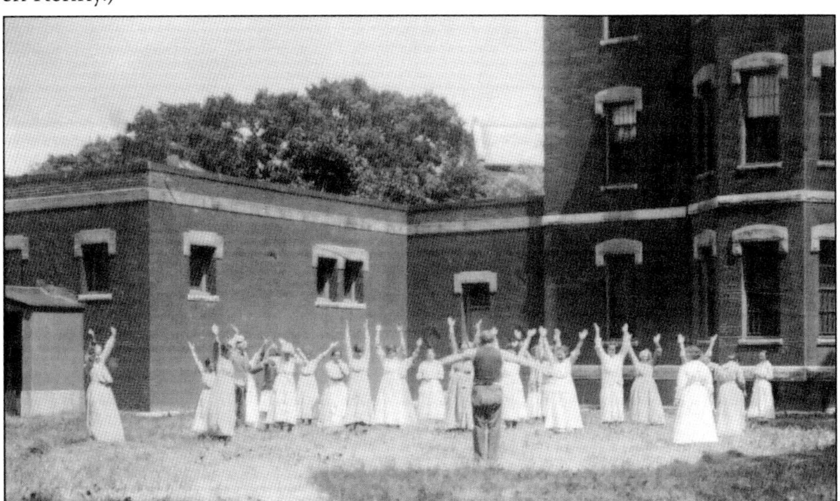

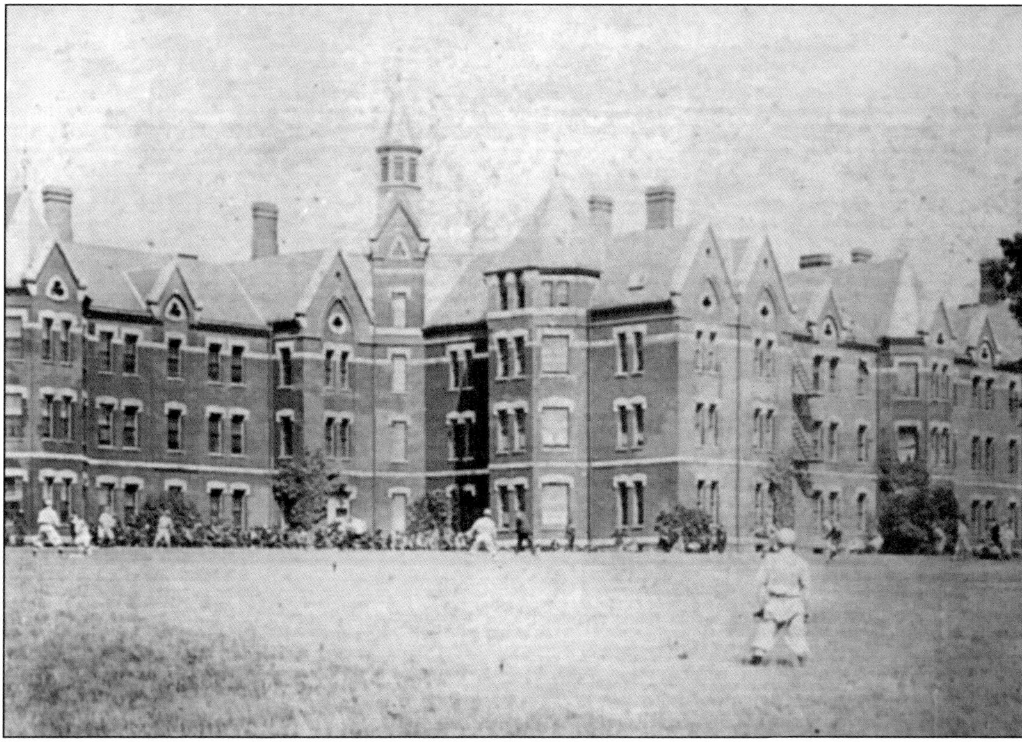

As part of their treatment, patients were often encouraged to participate in team activities to improve their social interactions. Here, patients team up for a baseball game on the front lawn organized by staff members. As can be seen in the photograph, the patient teams even had uniforms of their own. (John Gray.)

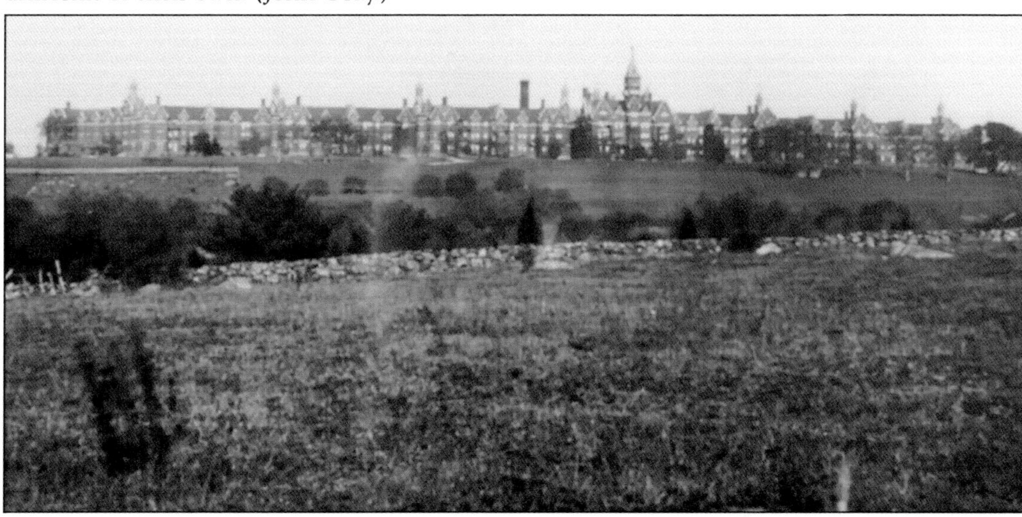

John Hathorne (son of William and grandfather of author Nathaniel Hawthorne) returned to his father's house on Hathorne Hill in 1692. He served as chief examiner in the Salem witch trials, one of the few who showed no remorse for contributing to the hysteria that swept New England. Author H.P. Lovecraft would eventually capitalize on that sordid reputation when creating his fictional Arkham. In his story "Pickman's Model," he even mentions the asylum by name. This glass-plate image is from around 1880. (Danvers Archival Center, Danvers, Massachusetts.)

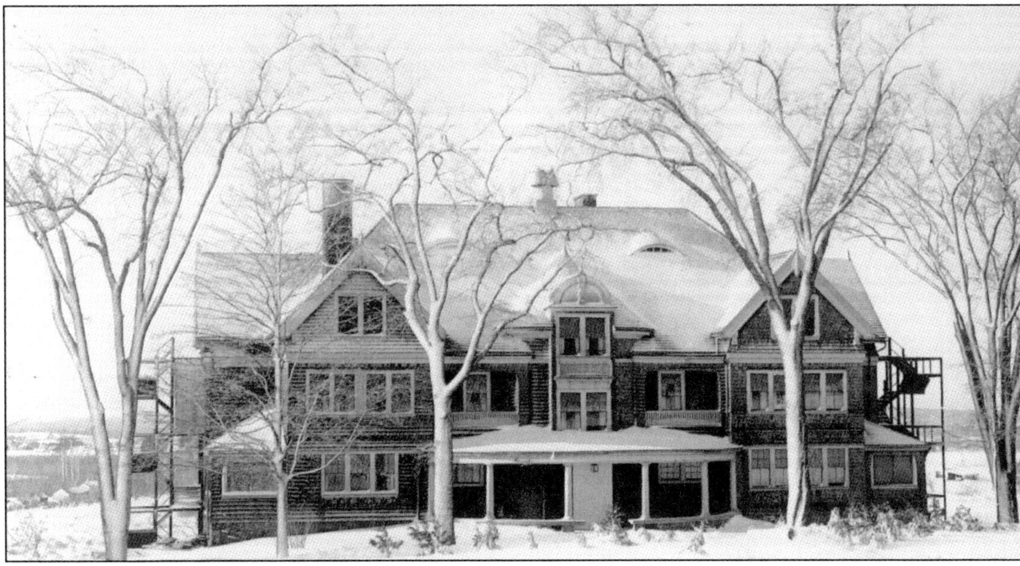

William Hathorne, a puritan judge who came to the New World in 1630, was as notorious as his son John, having ordered the public whipping of a Quaker woman in 1662. In order to begin construction, Hathorne's mansion atop the hill had to be demolished. When it was, the ornate doorknocker was saved and later added to the front door of Gray Gables, the nurses' cottage constructed in 1898. Gray Gables sat slightly below the main hospital building and would be dismantled with the first wave of demolition after the hospital's closure. (Above, Danvers Archival Center, Danvers, Massachusetts; below, John Gray.)

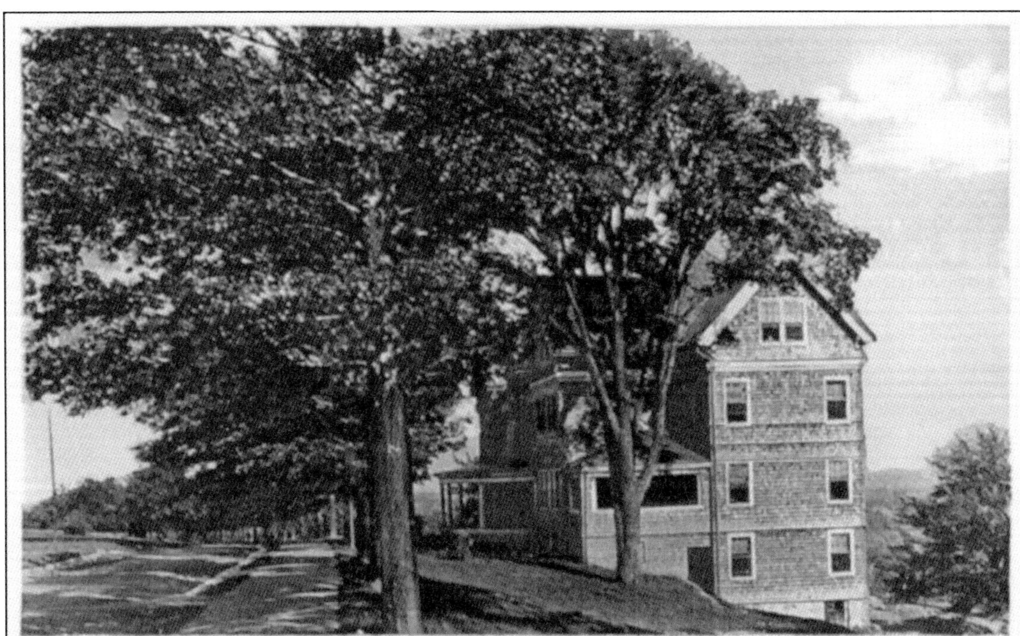

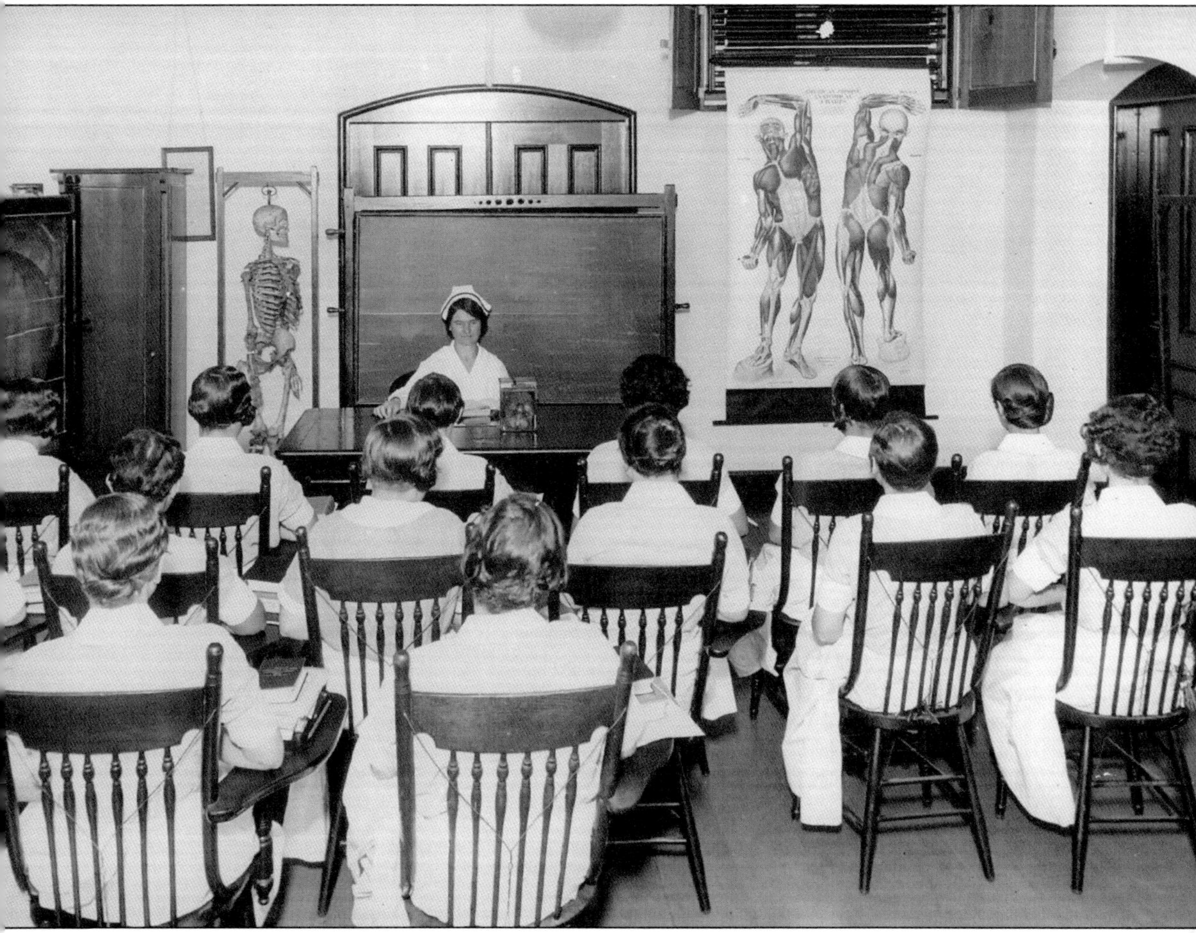

In 1889, Danvers State Hospital established the second nursing school in Massachusetts as well as the second nurses' home (Gray Gables). A principal was appointed to the school, and a rotating series of lectures on psychiatric nursing were presented to the student nurses. (Danvers Archival Center, Danvers, Massachusetts.)

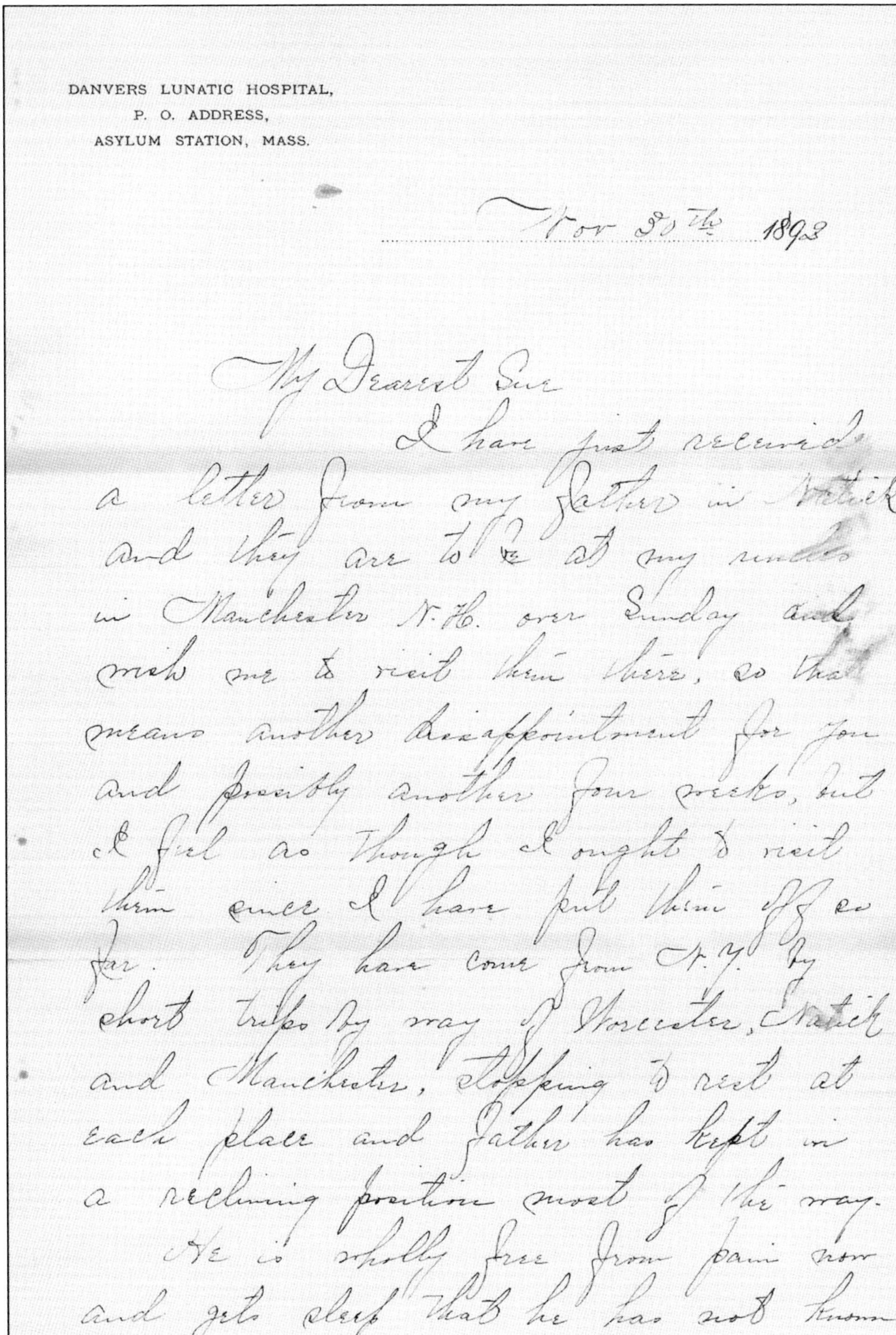
DANVERS LUNATIC HOSPITAL,
P. O. ADDRESS,
ASYLUM STATION, MASS.

Nov 30th 1893

My Dearest Sir

I have just received a letter from my father in Natick and they are to be at my uncles in Manchester N.H. over Sunday and wish me to visit them there, so that means another disappointment for you and possibly another four weeks, but I feel as though I ought to visit them since I have put them off so far. They have come from N.Y. by short trips by way of Worcester, Natick and Manchester, stopping to rest at each place and father has kept in a reclining position most of the way.

He is wholly free from pain now and gets sleep that he has not known

This letter, dated November 30, 1893, was written by an employee of the asylum and sent to a fellow employee at the Butler Hospital in Providence, Rhode Island. The letter goes on to speak of the daily activities on campus as well as the doctors' comings and goings. (Karen Bourdelais.)

Two

Expansion

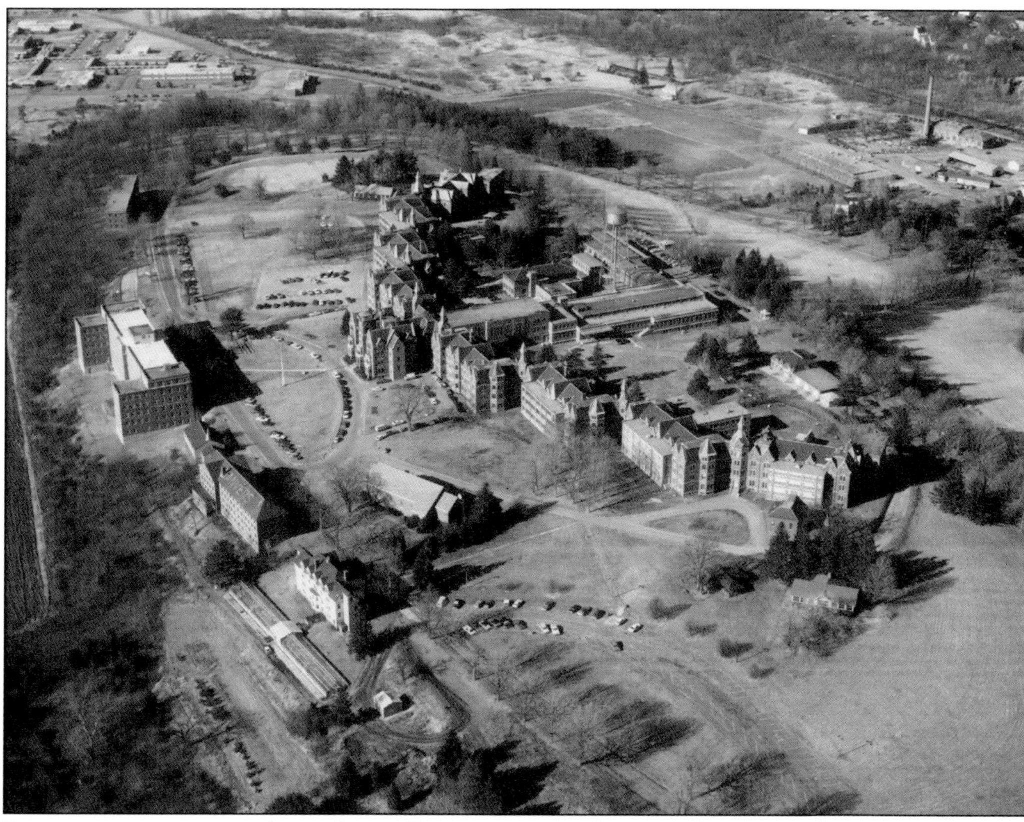

Danvers was constructed mainly to alleviate overcrowding in other Massachusetts institutions, but as early as 1901, the trustees were lamenting the pains of housing more than 1,000 patients in a hospital built for 450. The need for more funding and physical expansion was immediate, and Danvers began to stretch its wings across Hathorne Hill. (Massachusetts Archives.)

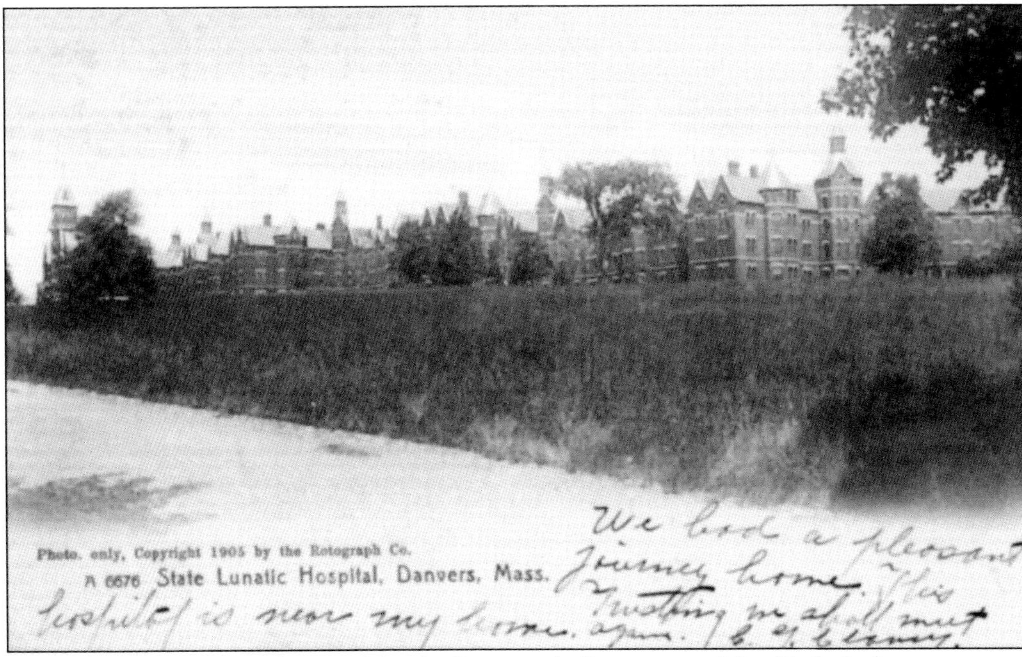

This postcard was printed in 1905 by the Rotograph Company in New York. It shows a view of the main administration tower and the female wing of the hospital. The message reads, "We had a pleasant journey home. This hospital is near my home. Trusting we shall meet again." (Ethan Dexter.)

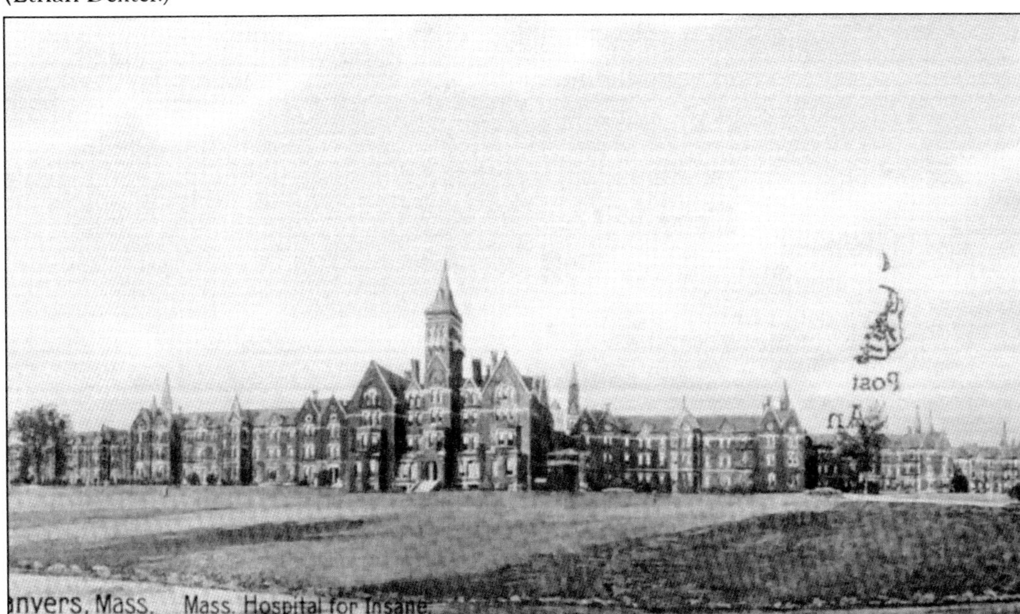

Another early postcard of the asylum, this one in full color, shows a front view of the hospital from the drive up Hathorne Hill. Asylum postcards such as these were very popular for visitors to send well into the early 20th century. Eventually, nearly every asylum in the United States would have its own postcard. Some, like Danvers and its sister institution in Worcester, would have hundreds. (Ethan Dexter.)

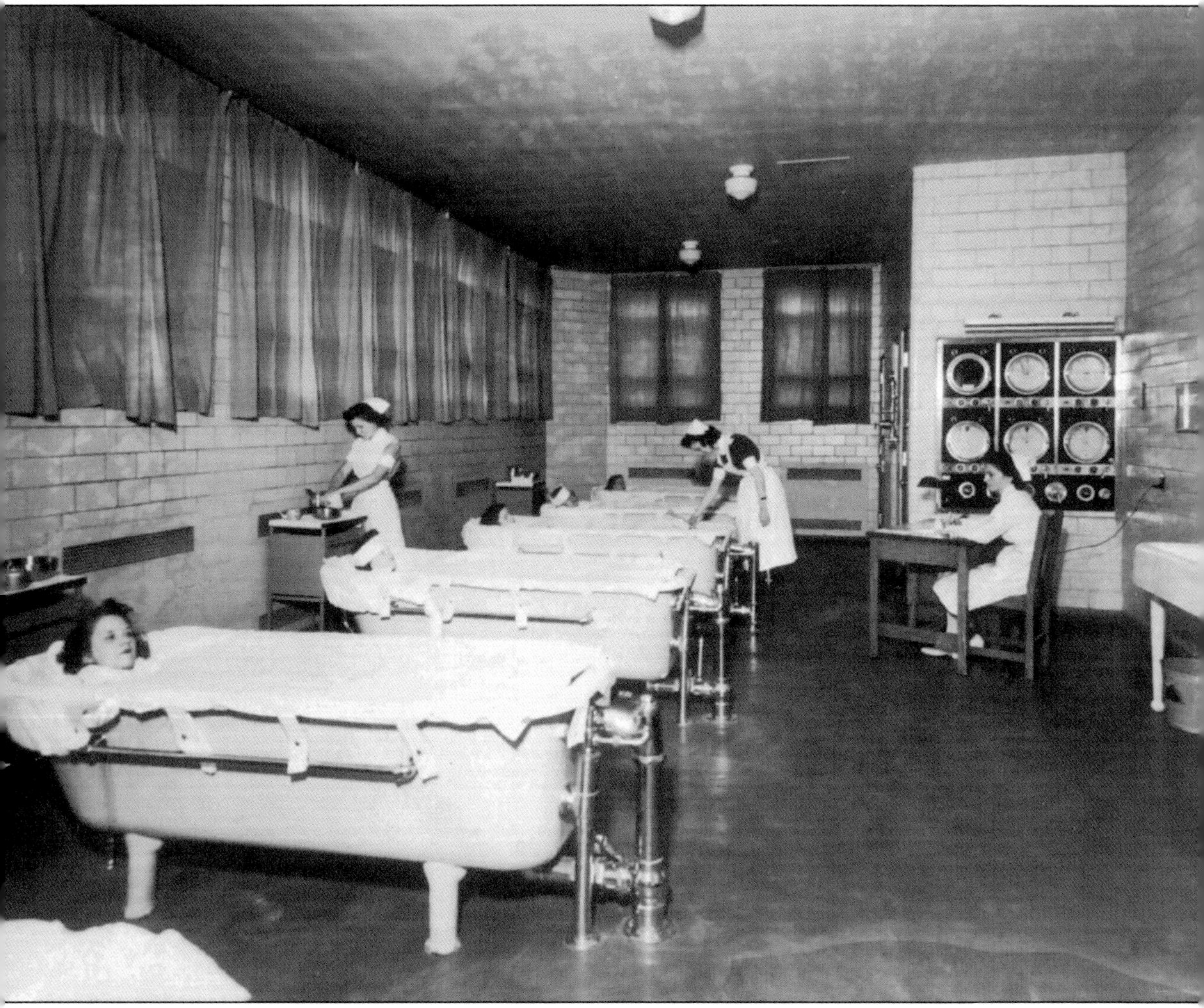

Hydrotherapy, also called the "water cure," became a primary ingredient in the treatment program at Danvers, along with recreational therapy, occupational therapy, and fresh air. Originally offered in stand-alone clinics, hydrotherapy was first introduced into asylums in 1866 at Battle Creek Sanitarium. It was believed that the use of water baths could treat the "clogged condition of the brain" more effectively than restraints of drugs and could be accomplished with baths, packs, or sprays. Warm continuous baths were used to treat insomnia and calm agitation. A patient could expect a continuous bath treatment to last anywhere from several hours to several days in water temperatures ranging from 92 degrees to 97 degrees Fahrenheit. Packs consisted of sheets dipped in varying temperatures of water, wrapped around the patient. Hydrotherapy at Danvers was so successful that two separate hydrotherapy units were built to the rear of Wards B and I in 1926. (Ben Kenny.)

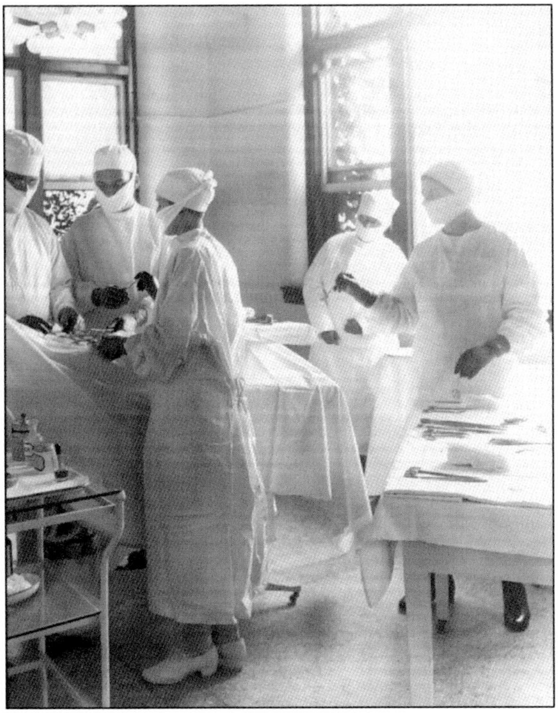

Electroconvulsive therapy, or shock therapy as it is commonly known, was introduced as a treatment for mental illness in 1938. Used to treat primarily major depressive disorders, its use was limited to carefully selected cases at Danvers State Hospital, though psychosurgery was common at the asylum. Weekly medical and surgical rounds were made on all wards, but eventually, it became clear that there was a need for a separate surgical unit that would also contain an isolation wing. Later, the surgical services would be moved to the Bonner Building, where they would remain until the hospital closed. (Left, Ben Kenny; below, John Gray.)

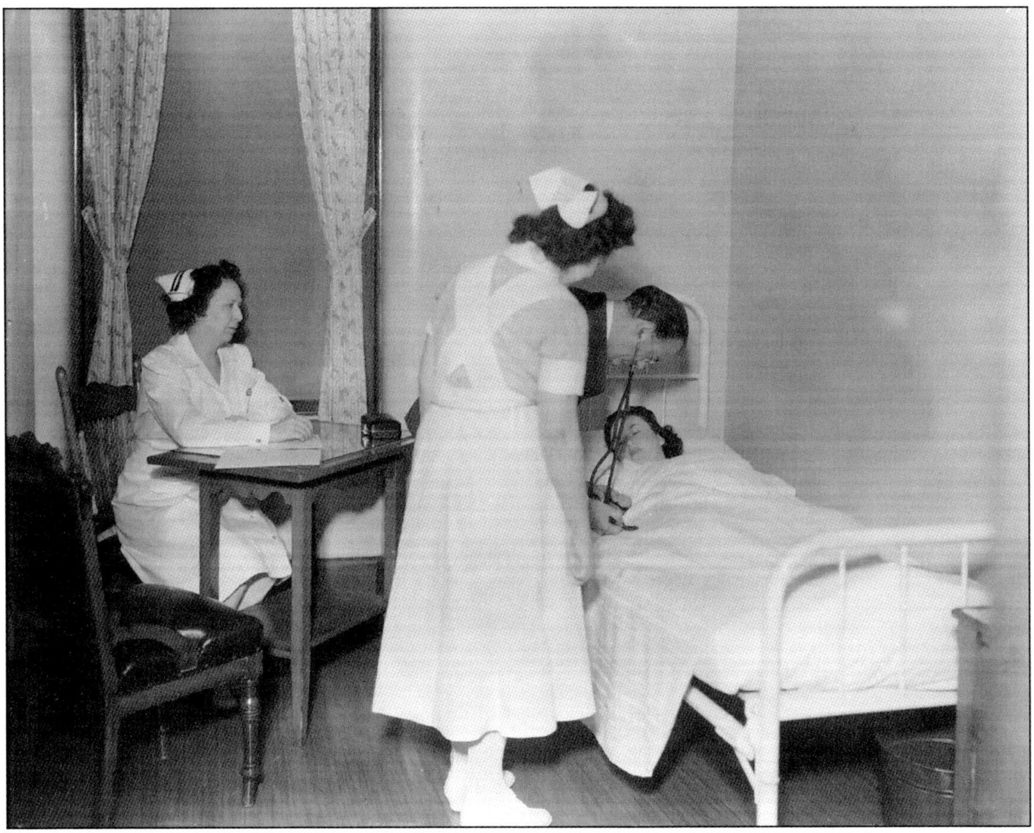

Very often, advances in the care of the mentally ill were touted as "wonders" or "miracles"—cure-alls that were often presented as such to the general public. Hoping to combat the assumption that these miracles existed, the DSH Auxiliary called simply for good science and continued humane patient treatment. New treatments and medications often complicated care further and certainly did not alleviate the plague of overcrowding and lack of adequate funding. At times, staff morale was quite low, as evidenced by this resignation letter penned by a worker who was dissatisfied with the ward supervisor's methods. (Right, John Gray; below, David Walsh.)

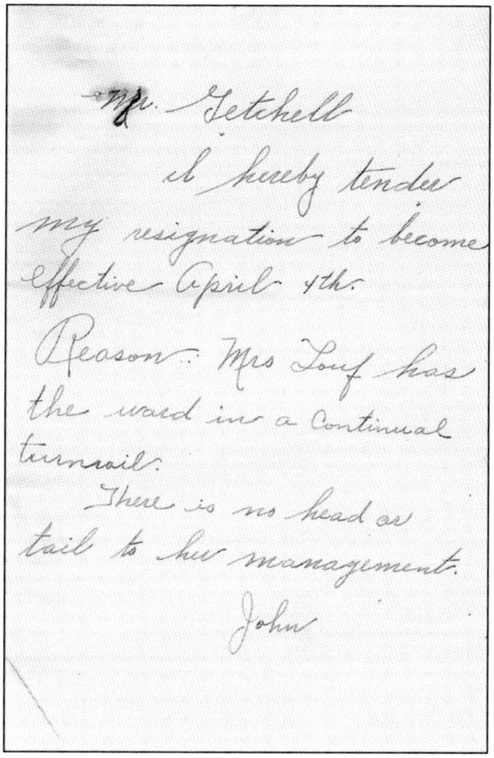

Mr. Getchell

I hereby tender my resignation to become effective April 4th.

Reason: Mrs Louf has the ward in a continual turmoil.

There is no head or tail to her management.

John

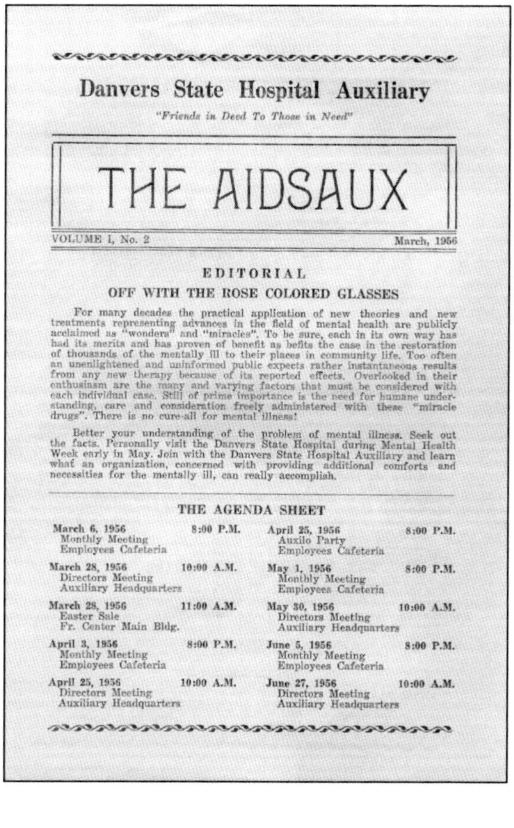

Danvers State Hospital Auxiliary

"Friends in Deed To Those in Need"

THE AIDSAUX

VOLUME I, No. 2 — March, 1956

EDITORIAL

OFF WITH THE ROSE COLORED GLASSES

For many decades the practical application of new theories and new treatments representing advances in the field of mental health are publicly acclaimed as "wonders" and "miracles". To be sure, each in its own way has had its merits and has proven of benefit as befits the case in the restoration of thousands of the mentally ill to their places in community life. Too often an unenlightened and uninformed public expects rather instantaneous results from any new therapy because of its reported effects. Overlooked in their enthusiasm are the many and varying factors that must be considered with each individual case. Still of prime importance is the need for humane understanding, care and consideration freely administered with these "miracle drugs". There is no cure-all for mental illness!

Better your understanding of the problem of mental illness. Seek out the facts. Personally visit the Danvers State Hospital during Mental Health Week early in May. Join with the Danvers State Hospital Auxiliary and learn what an organization, concerned with providing additional comforts and necessities for the mentally ill, can really accomplish.

THE AGENDA SHEET

March 6, 1956 — **8:00 P.M.**
Monthly Meeting
Employees Cafeteria

March 28, 1956 — **10:00 A.M.**
Directors Meeting
Auxiliary Headquarters

March 28, 1956 — **11:00 A.M.**
Easter Sale
Fr. Center Main Bldg.

April 3, 1956 — **8:00 P.M.**
Monthly Meeting
Employees Cafeteria

April 25, 1956 — **10:00 A.M.**
Directors Meeting
Auxiliary Headquarters

April 25, 1956 — **8:00 P.M.**
Auxilo Party
Employees Cafeteria

May 1, 1956 — **8:00 P.M.**
Monthly Meeting
Employees Cafeteria

May 30, 1956 — **10:00 A.M.**
Directors Meeting
Auxiliary Headquarters

June 5, 1956 — **8:00 P.M.**
Monthly Meeting
Employees Cafeteria

June 27, 1956 — **10:00 A.M.**
Directors Meeting
Auxiliary Headquarters

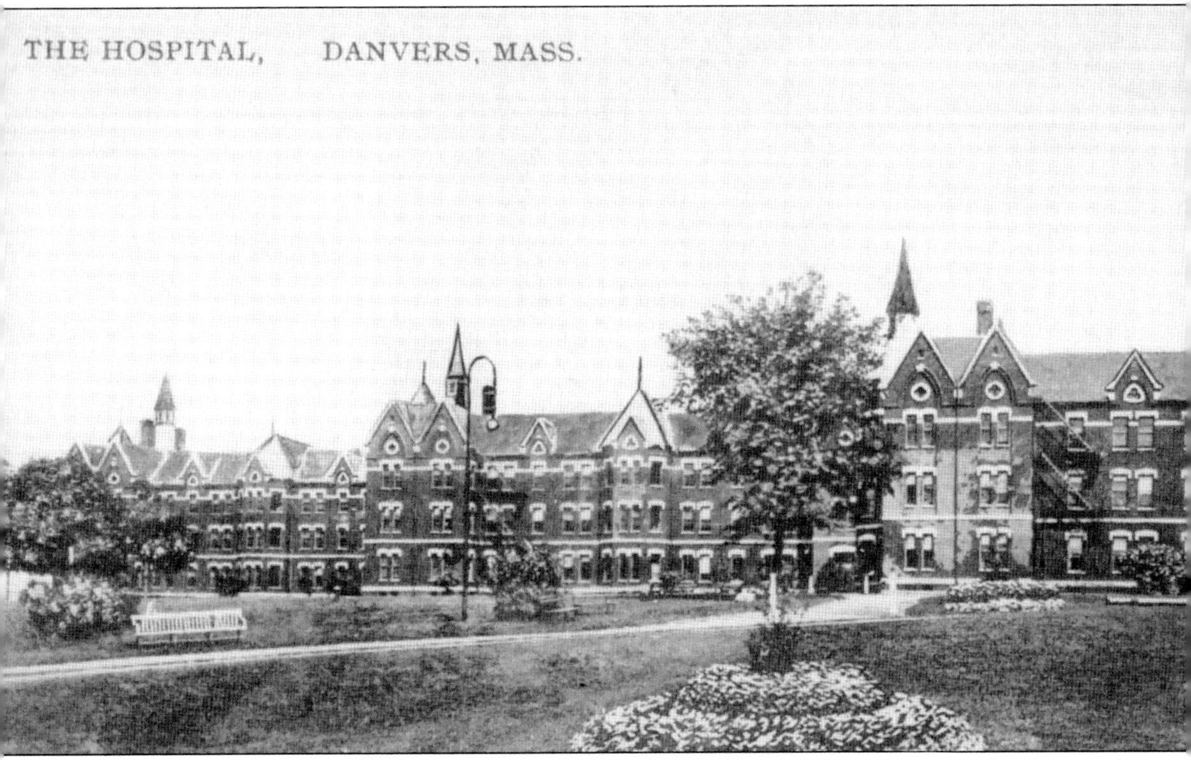

By the 1930s, numerous requests for repairs to the hospital were already being made. Fireproof staircases were added on the wards and all wiring was replaced. The sprinkler system in A and J buildings was updated, and the hospital was connected directly with the town's electric supply. In spite of these repairs, the trustees continued to lament the growing population and asked that

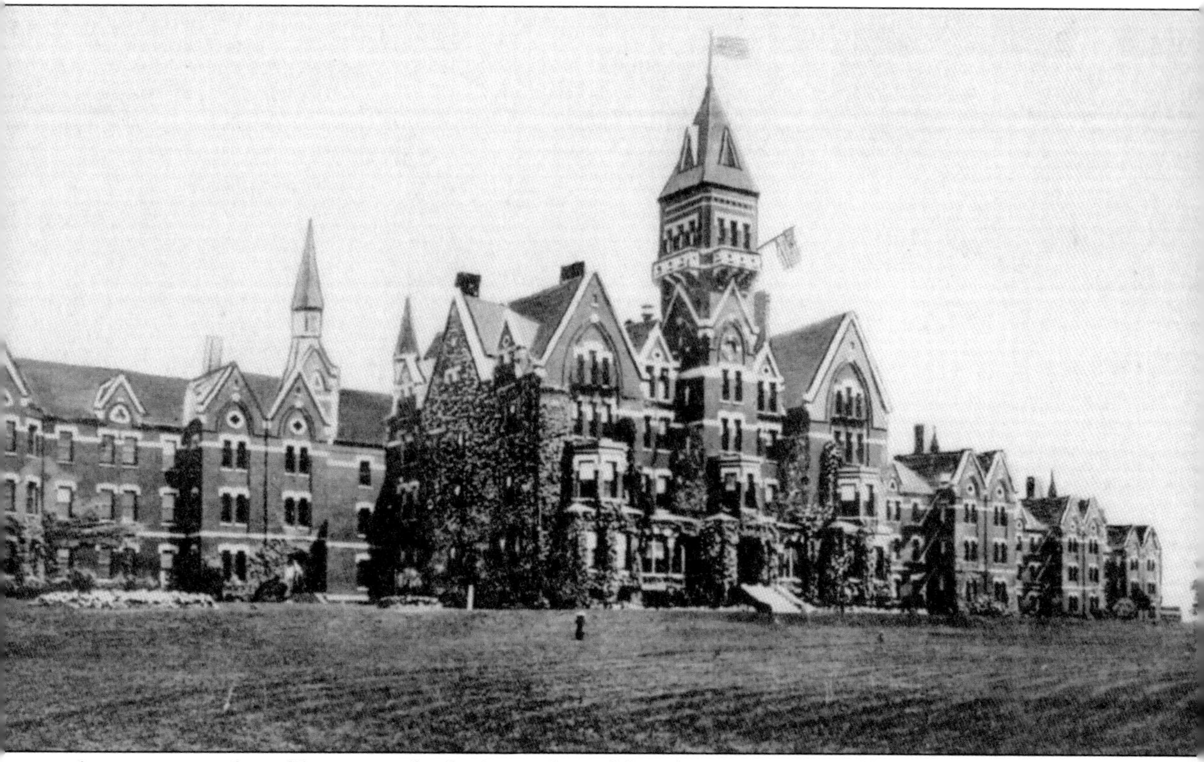

the state consider adding on to both the male and female sections, as well as adding a building solely for the care of tuberculosis patients. They also requested the addition of an acute reception building, meant to separate those patients from the chronic cases. (Taylor Raab.)

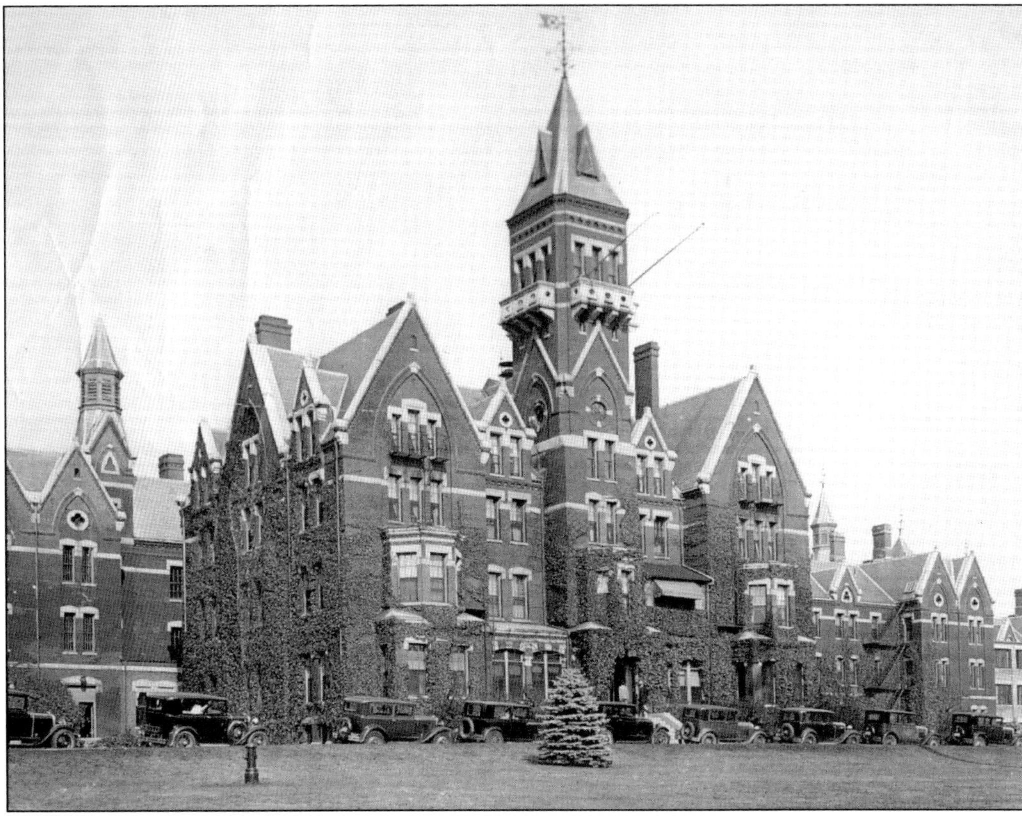

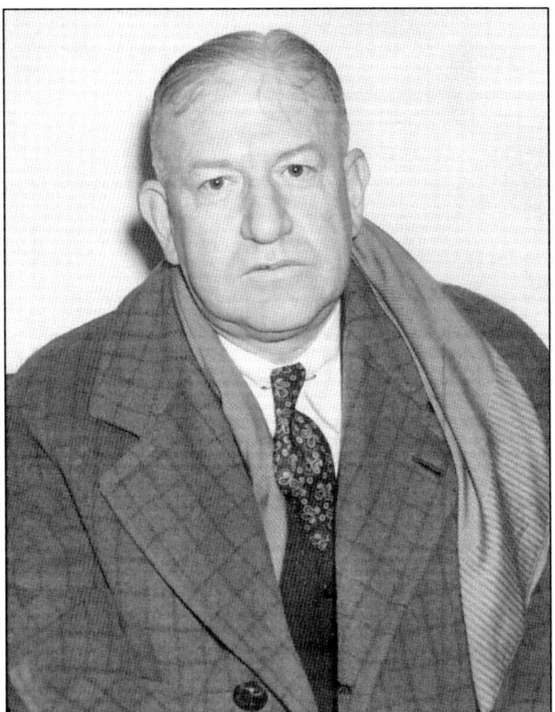

The 1935 annual report noted that the main hospital underwent a number of improvements. The wooden staircases in both the male and female wards were replaced by fireproof ones, wiring was updated, and water pressure was improved. The superintendent, Dr. Clarence Bonner, reported that the hydrotherapy units were being enlarged and that new equipment was installed, though wet sheet packs and continuous bath treatments were being used in the absence of the hydrotherapy units. An intensive study of the tuberculosis problem amongst the patients was undertaken, and the trustees requested that tuberculosis units be constructed on campus. Continued lectures were given to nursing staff throughout Essex County in a number of disciplines. (Above, Danvers Archival Center, Danvers, Massachusetts; left, John Gray.)

In 1937, the federally funded Works Progress Association helped to complete painting. The new hydrotherapy buildings opened, and the physiotherapy department began incorporating massage and light treatments into the patients' care. On February 18, 1937, Dr. Peter Hagopian was appointed assistant physician under Clarence Bonner. He would serve in that role until taking over for Bonner upon his retirement in 1954. (John Gray.)

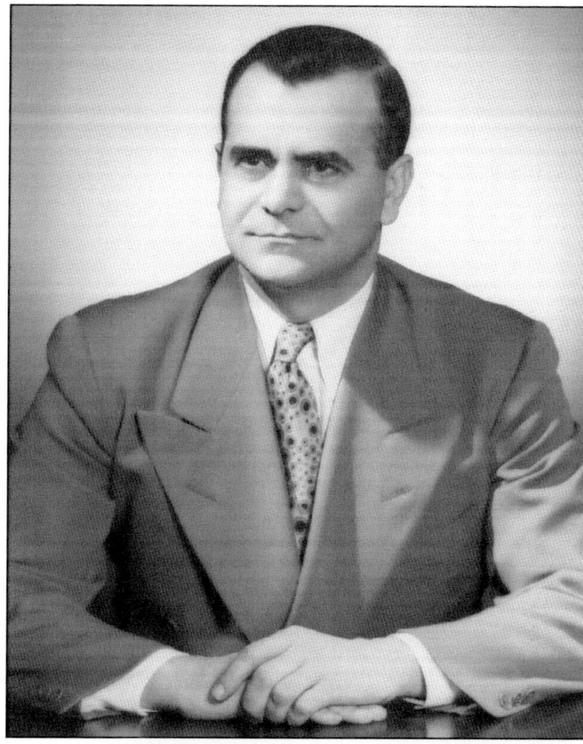

By the time the hospital trustees issued their annual report for 1940, the hospital was serving more than 2,400 patients, causing serious overcrowding. The Department of Mental Health alleviated some of the overcrowding through transfers and redistricting, requiring cities to begin sending patients to Worcester State Hospital instead. (David Walsh.)

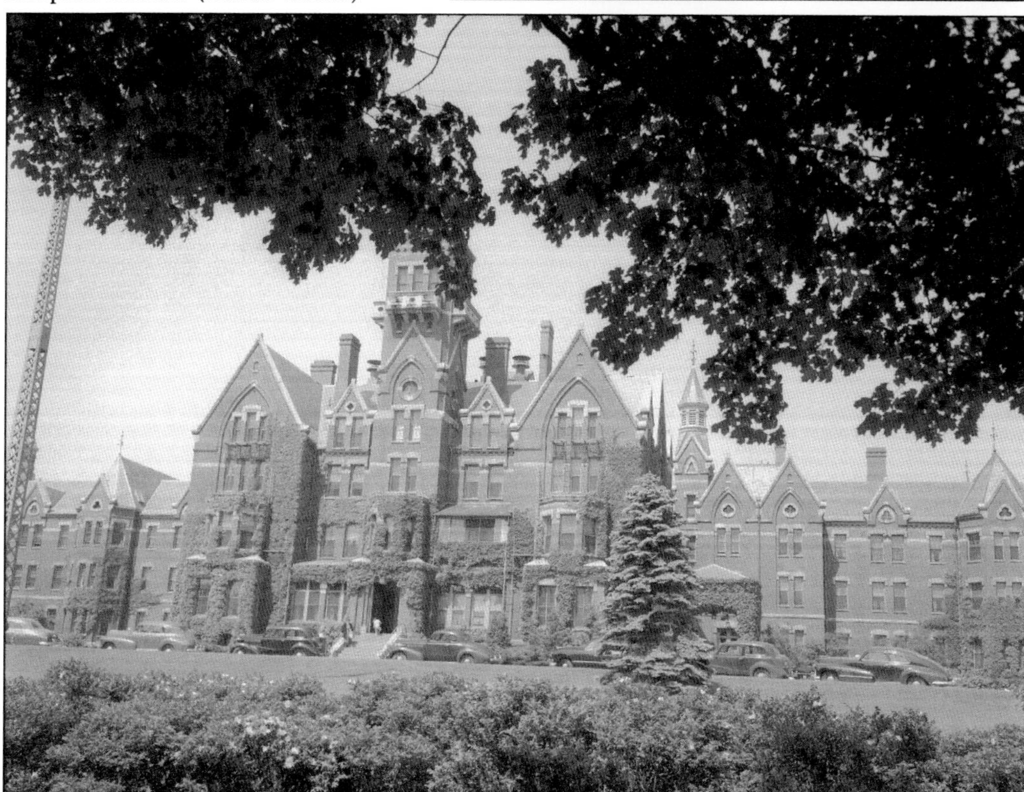

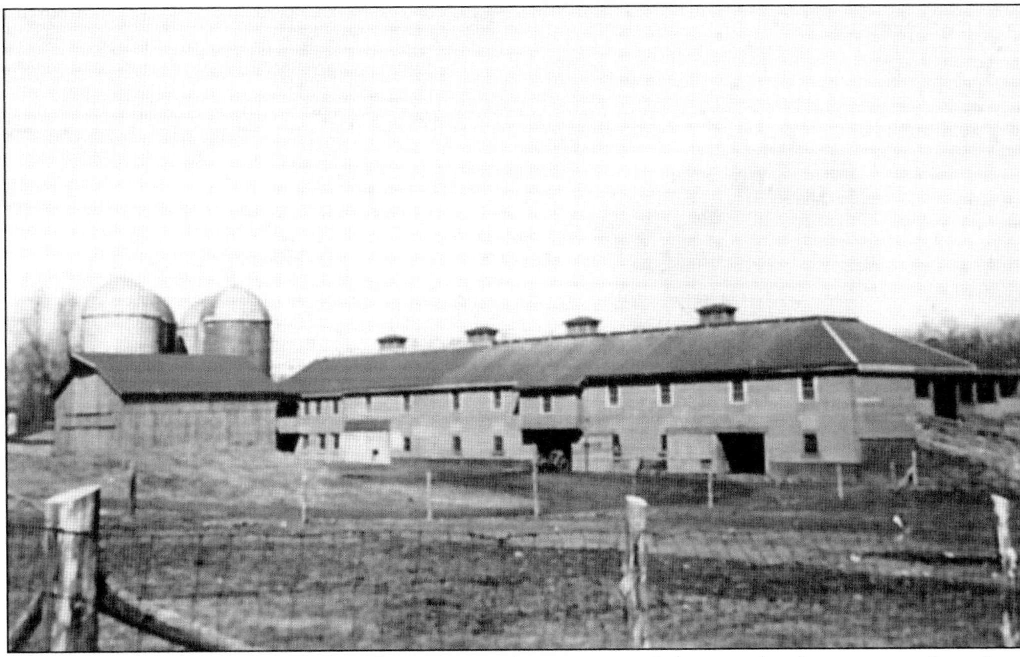

The state hospital farm was not only a source of occupational therapy for the patients, but also a major producer of all the food the state hospital needed including eggs, beef, pork, and poultry. The gardens grew nearly all the produce used in the kitchens and became well known for the "Danvers onion." In the early 1930s, a drought severely decimated the crops. The cows suffered from infectious mastitis, which lessened the milk supply. The hay production was also severely impacted by the drought, but later farm reports noted that the farm was able to recover and the yield returned to normal. (John Gray.)

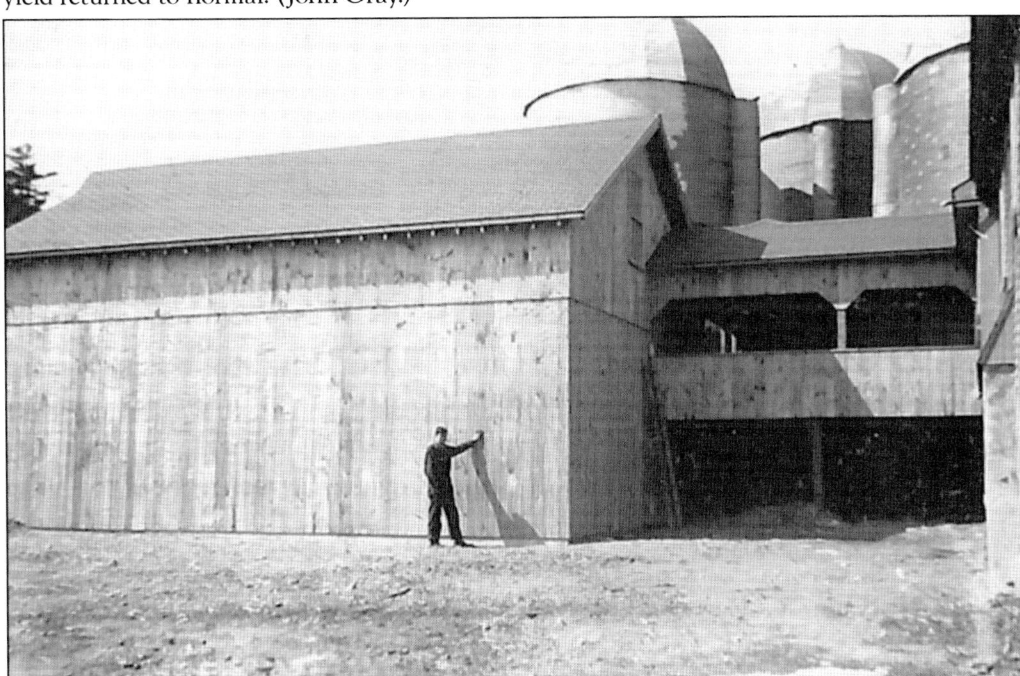

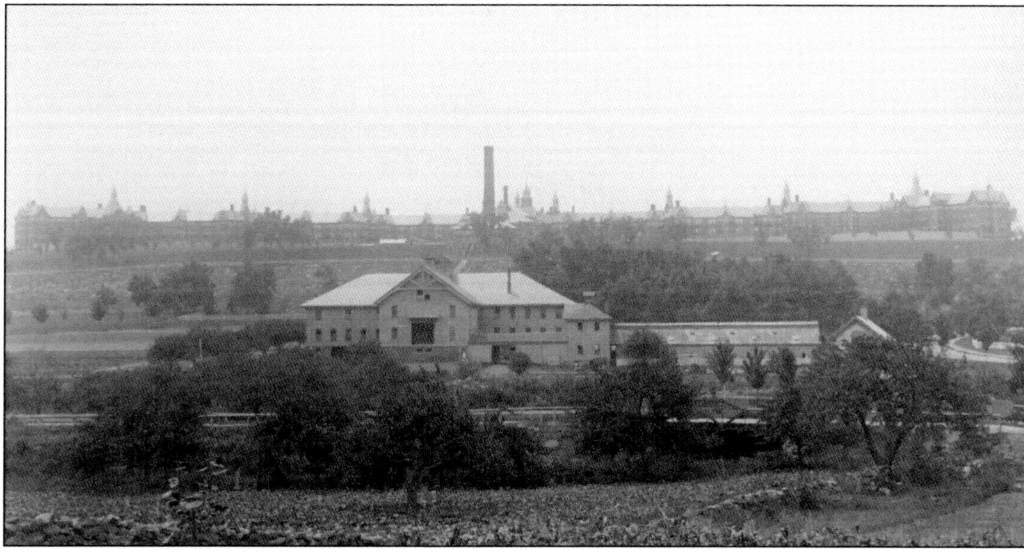

This 1884 view of the state hospital shows the farm to the rear of the Kirkbride, with the power house and pump house in the distance. Absent from the image are Farm Hall and Grove Hall, which were added in 1902 and 1931, respectively. (Danvers Archival Center, Danvers, Massachusetts.)

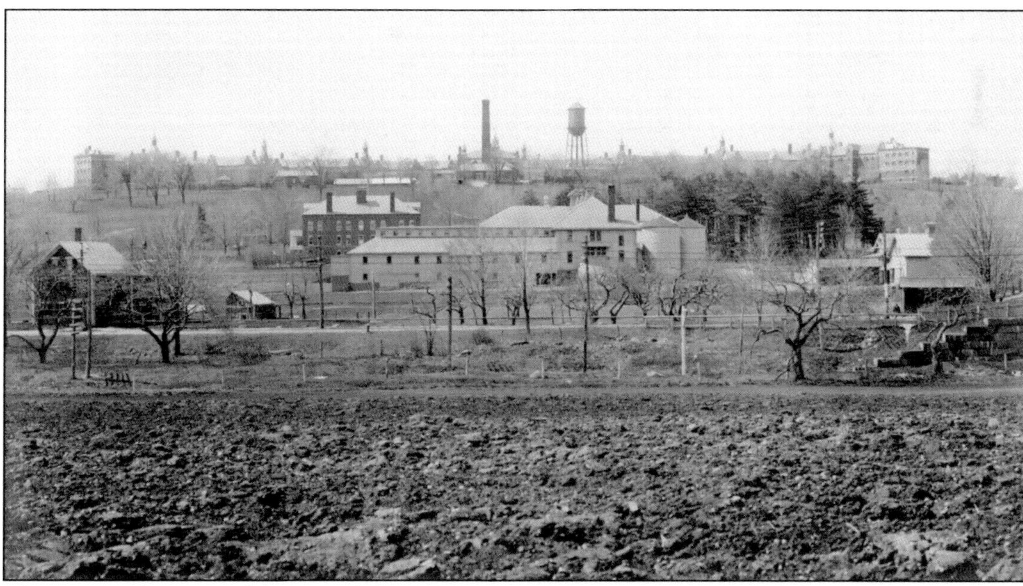

This is a similar view of the rear of the Kirkbride in the 1920s. Note the addition of the water tower, two grain silos, and, most notably, electricity. In the foreground, Grove Hall and a number of garages and maintenance buildings can be seen. (Danvers Archival Center, Danvers, Massachusetts.)

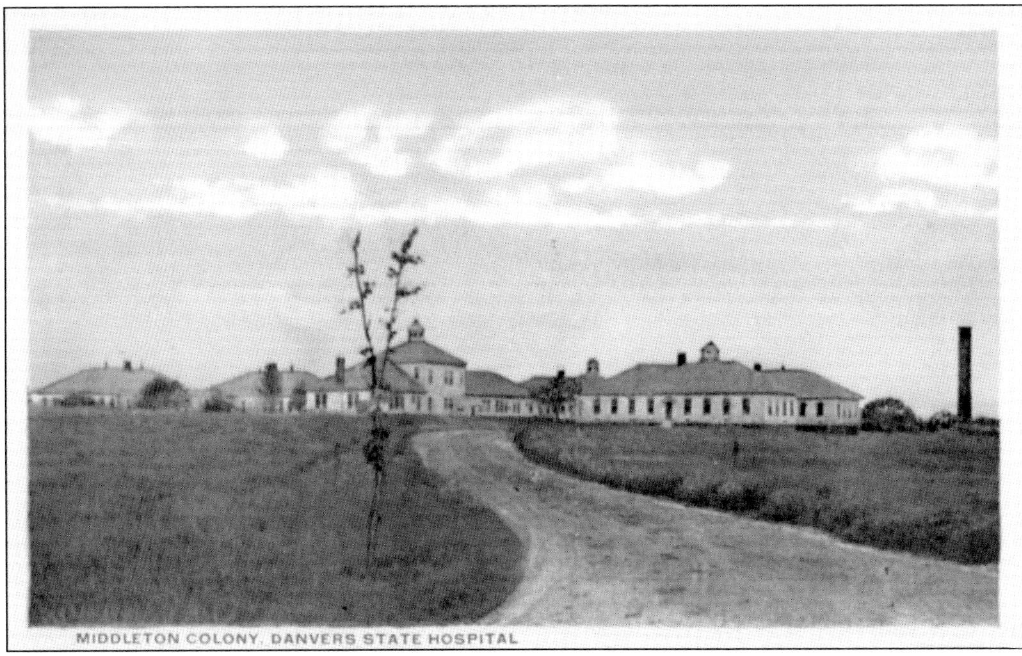

In 1902, Danvers State Hospital acquired another 100 acres, which straddled the towns of Danvers and Middleton. Major construction was undertaken, and a number of additions were built in 1903 to service the hospital farm—one of which was Middleton Colony, for female chronic patients. The farm had been in operation since the hospital's opening and had a piggery, corn barn, wagon shed, manure cellar, and apple orchards. With this expansion, large barns were built as housing for the men working the farm. The farm would become a "famous model," continuing to expand well into the 20th century. (Above, John Gray; below, Massachusetts Archives.)

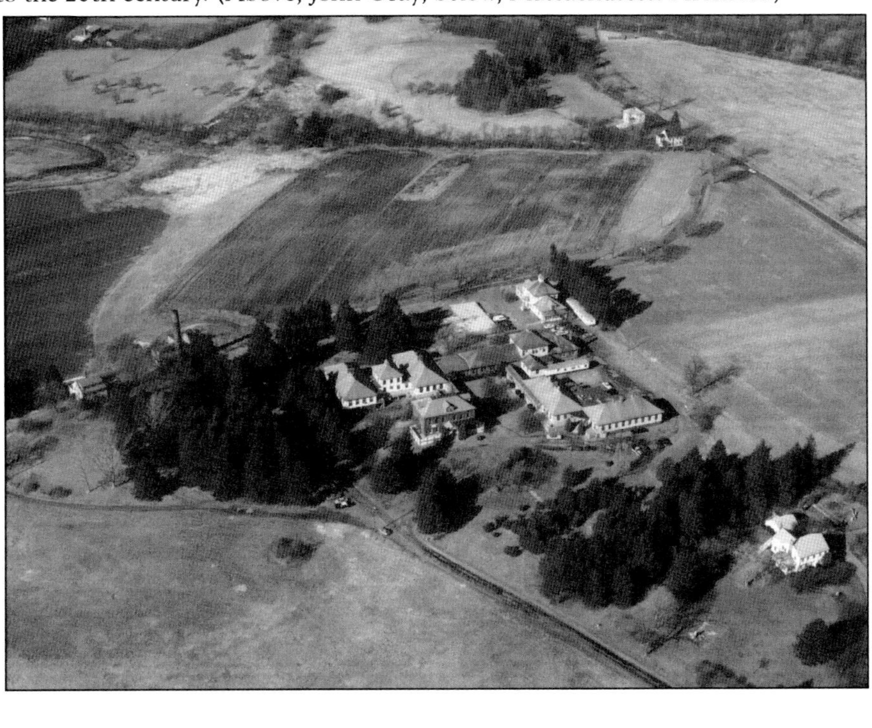

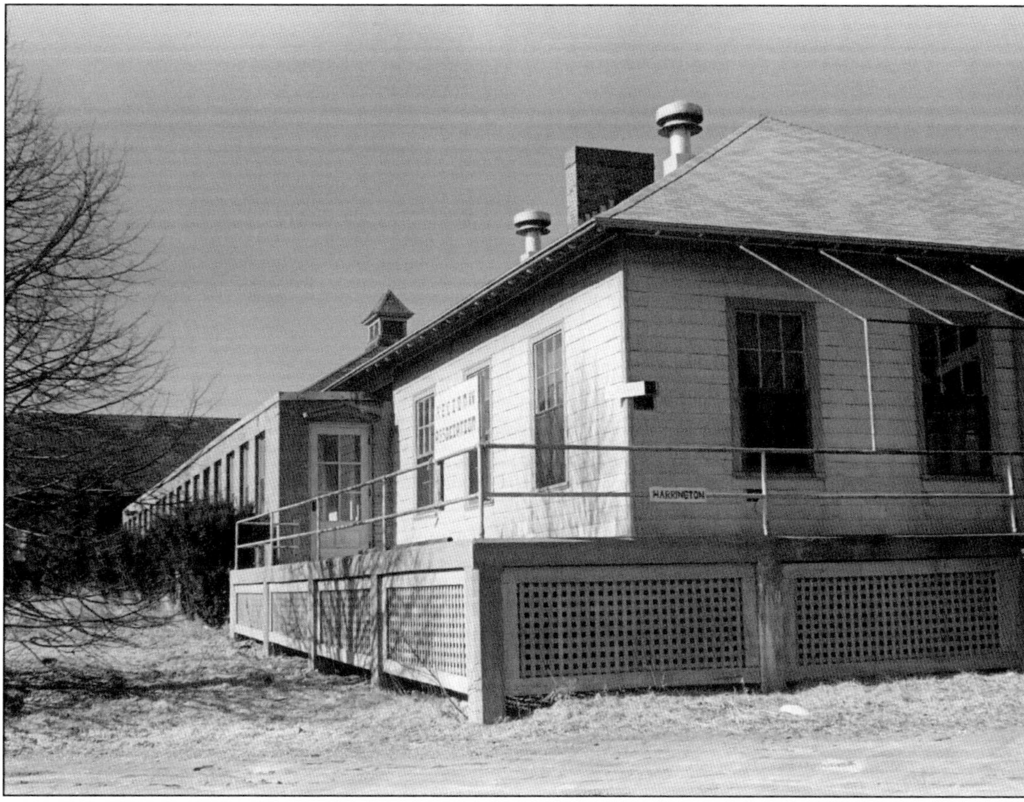

Also located on the lowlands were a number of farm cottages; some of which dated back to 1850, prior to the construction of the main hospital. By 1932, there was a total of six cottages. Some served as storage, with others as laundry and housing. A number of garages were added in the early 1950s, including a tractor shed, farm garage, implement shed, and a hay barn. Farm Hall would also later be added to the lowlands. Eventually, the new, more modern laundry building was added to the lowlands in 1965. The silos pictured here were added sometime prior to 1920. (Massachusetts Archives.)

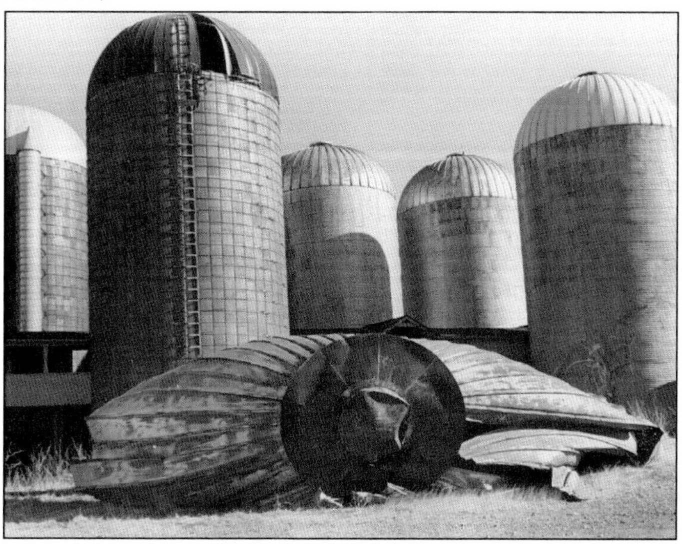

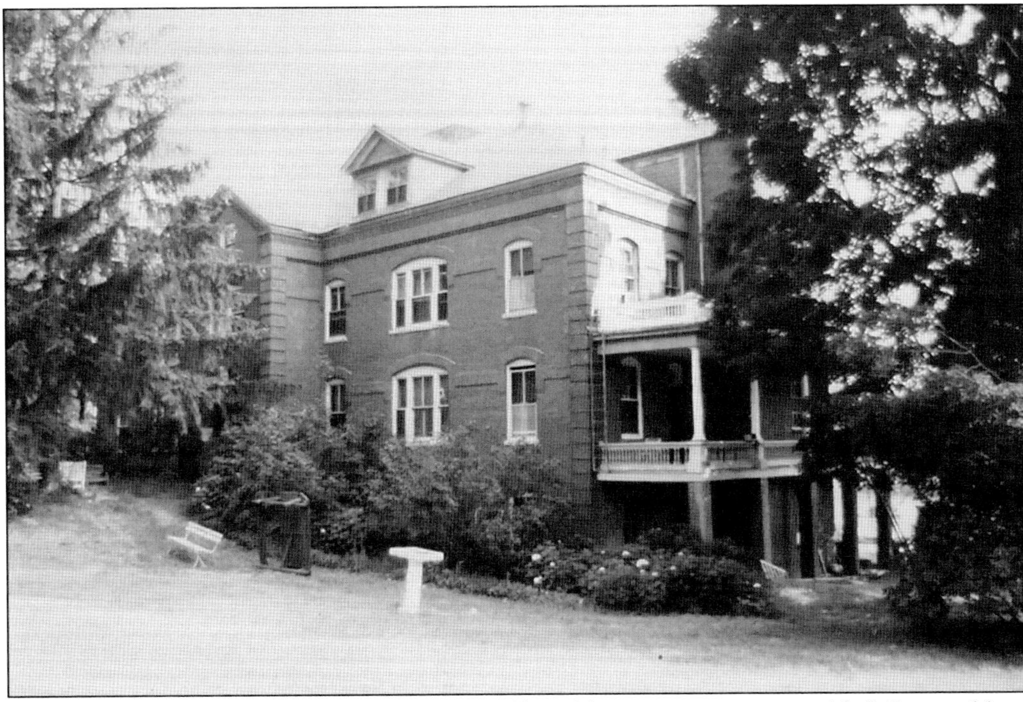

As the farm expanded, so too did the farm staff, and living quarters were added. Pictured here are Grove Hall, built in 1902, and Farm Hall was added in 1931, both housing male farm staff. The farm remained in operation well into the 1960s, including the slaughterhouse and the dairy where milk was processed. The asylum continued to grow its own fruits and vegetables, some of which were sent to the inmates at the Lawrence and Salem Jails. Grove Hall would later be converted into the Danvers Detox facility, while the Middleton Farm Colony would later house elderly patients. (Both, John Gray.)

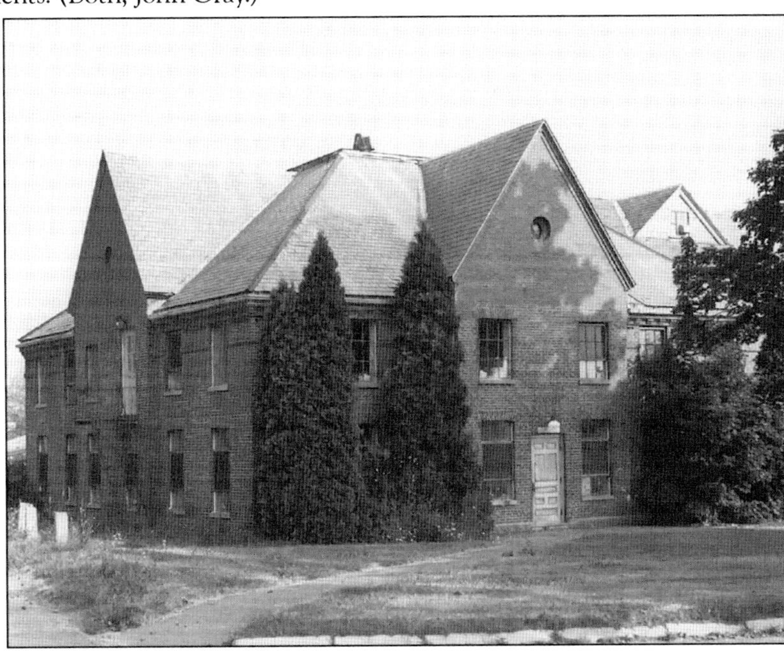

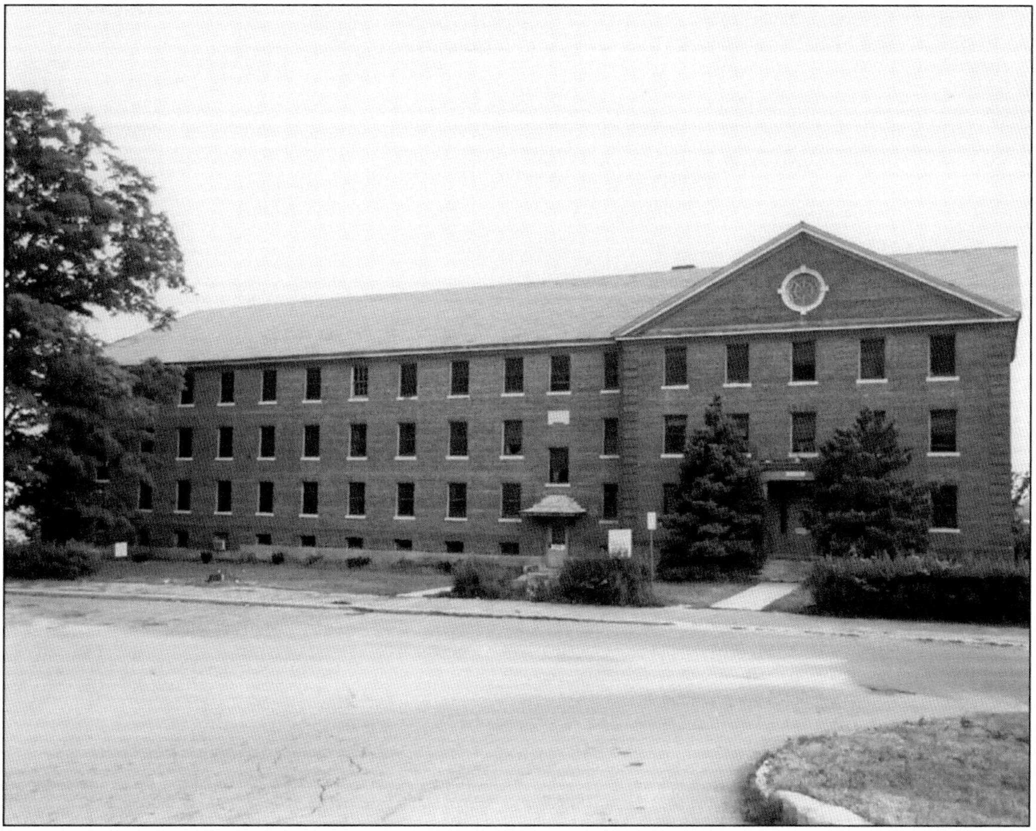

As the patient population at Danvers expanded, so too did the nursing staff. Gray Gables alone could no longer accommodate the number of nurses living on the grounds. The state hospital's nursing school continued to turn out graduates, of whom Superintendent Page had said that the intellectual and social status of nurses would be raised through better education. Two additional nurses' homes were added on either side of the hill, with one for male nurses in 1927 and one next door to Gray Gables for females in 1930. (Above, John Gray; right, Danvers Archival Center, Danvers, Massachusetts.)

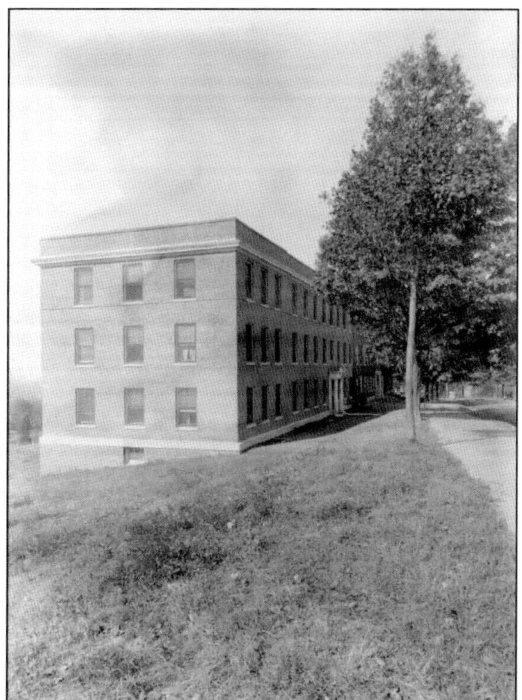

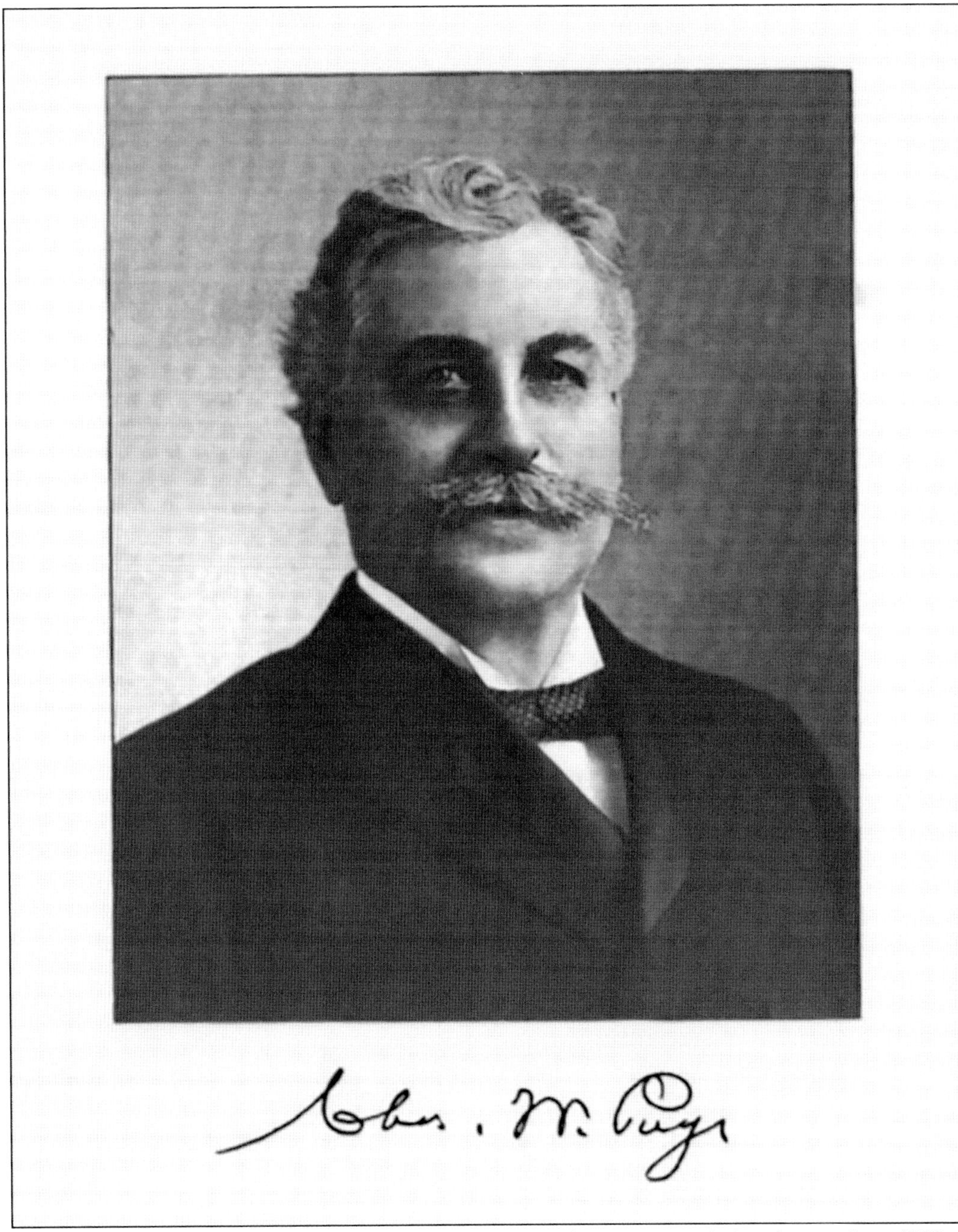

Dr. Charles Whitney Page, who served as superintendent from 1888 to 1898 and again from 1903 to 1910, developed the pathology department into one that gained national recognition. He assigned the first regular pathologist, Dr. William Leonard Worcester, in 1895, and they began the work of studying the brain tissue of patients in relation to their diagnosis, believing that there must be a clear biological cause for insanity. By the late 1880s, heredity was now listed as a possible cause for the admittance of some patients. Page was so progressive in his pursuit of a top-tier pathology laboratory that he even appointed women to the laboratory staff—a practice unheard of in many other institutions. (Katherine Anderson.)

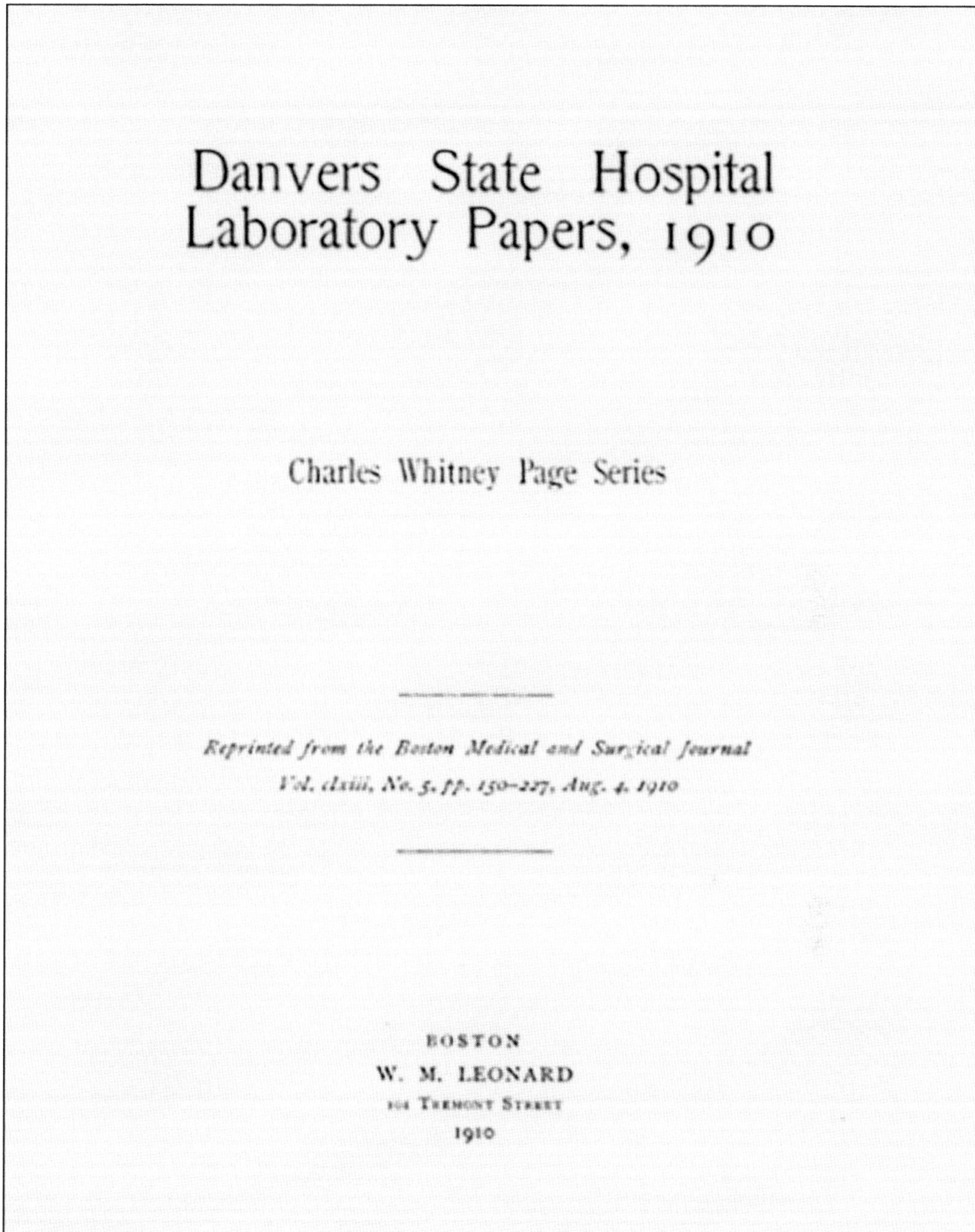

Danvers State Hospital
Laboratory Papers, 1910

Charles Whitney Page Series

Reprinted from the Boston Medical and Surgical Journal
Vol. clxiii, No. 5, pp. 150–227, Aug. 4, 1910

BOSTON
W. M. LEONARD
[illegible] TREMONT STREET
1910

Danvers State Hospital was well known for its cutting-edge pathology lab where doctors amassed a collection of brain tissue from each patient autopsied at the state hospital; the first of which was performed in 1879. In the first four months of Charles Whitney Page's tenure as superintendent, 61 patients died in hospital, 19 of whom underwent postmortem examinations. Page also noted in his first report as superintendent that the hospital continued in its practice of limiting the use of restraint, as well as continued to house patients on open wards. In 1910, the laboratory staff honored Page's departure from the superintendency by assembling every laboratory case from his tenure and publishing it publicly. (Katherine Anderson.)

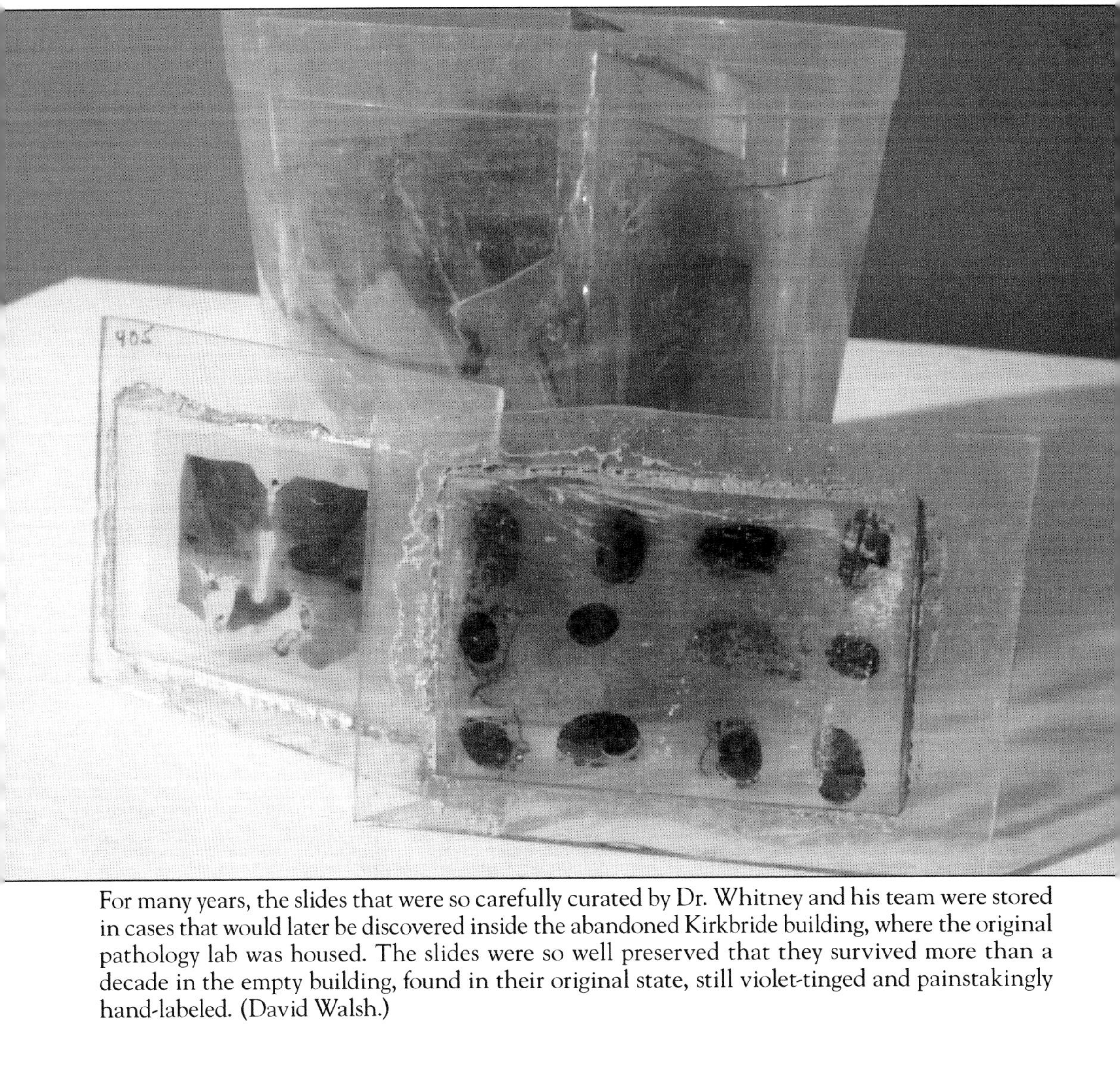

For many years, the slides that were so carefully curated by Dr. Whitney and his team were stored in cases that would later be discovered inside the abandoned Kirkbride building, where the original pathology lab was housed. The slides were so well preserved that they survived more than a decade in the empty building, found in their original state, still violet-tinged and painstakingly hand-labeled. (David Walsh.)

New pathology quarters were built behind the central administration building. Pathologists such as Dr. James J. Putnam and Dr. Sanger Brown built the asylum's specimen library and studied the brain tissue of patients to determine the root cause of many of the patients' illnesses. After the brains were photographed or cut up for autopsy, samples were taken from various regions of the brain, labeled, and then stained in Cresyl violet. Nearly 100 autopsies per year were performed at the state hospital. These slides were maintained in the pathology laboratory until the hospital's closing. (Right, David Walsh; below, John Gray.)

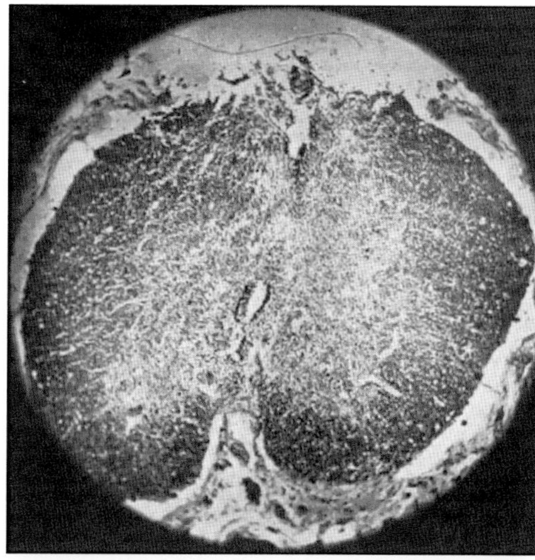

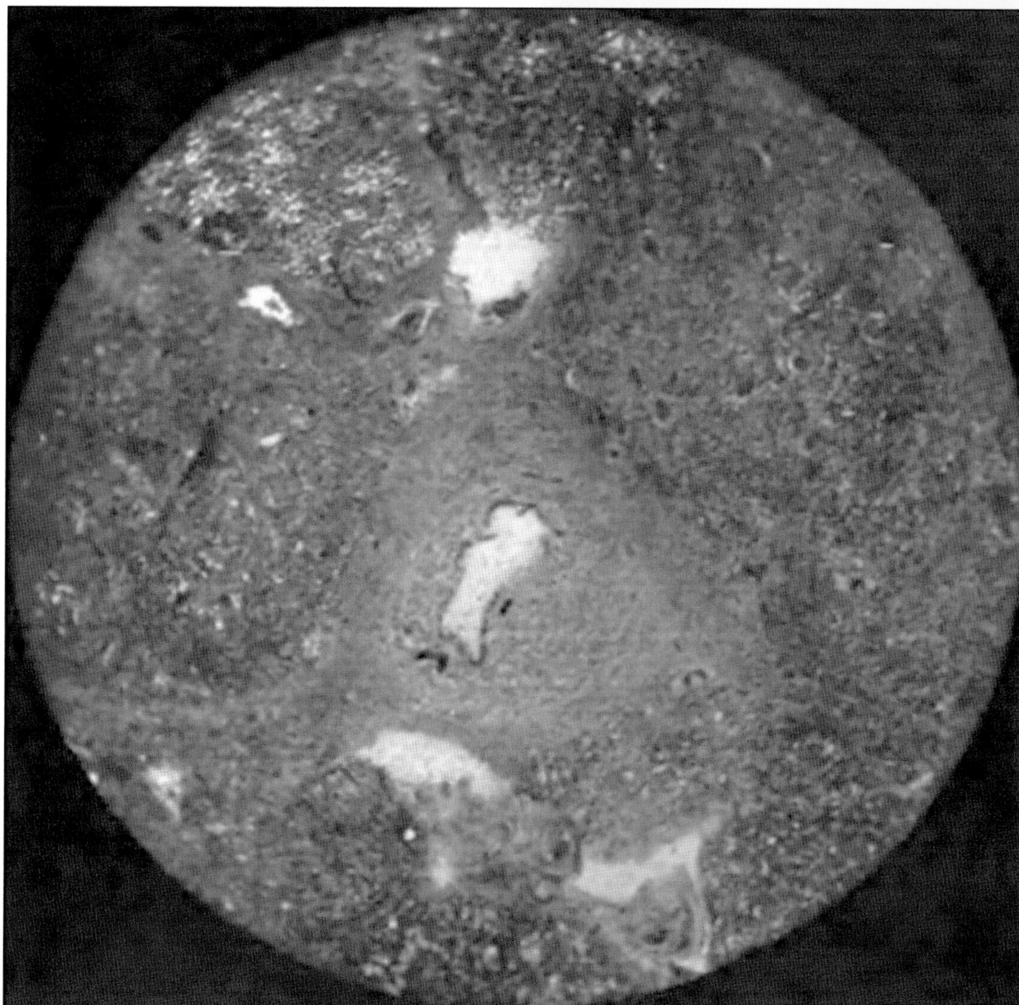

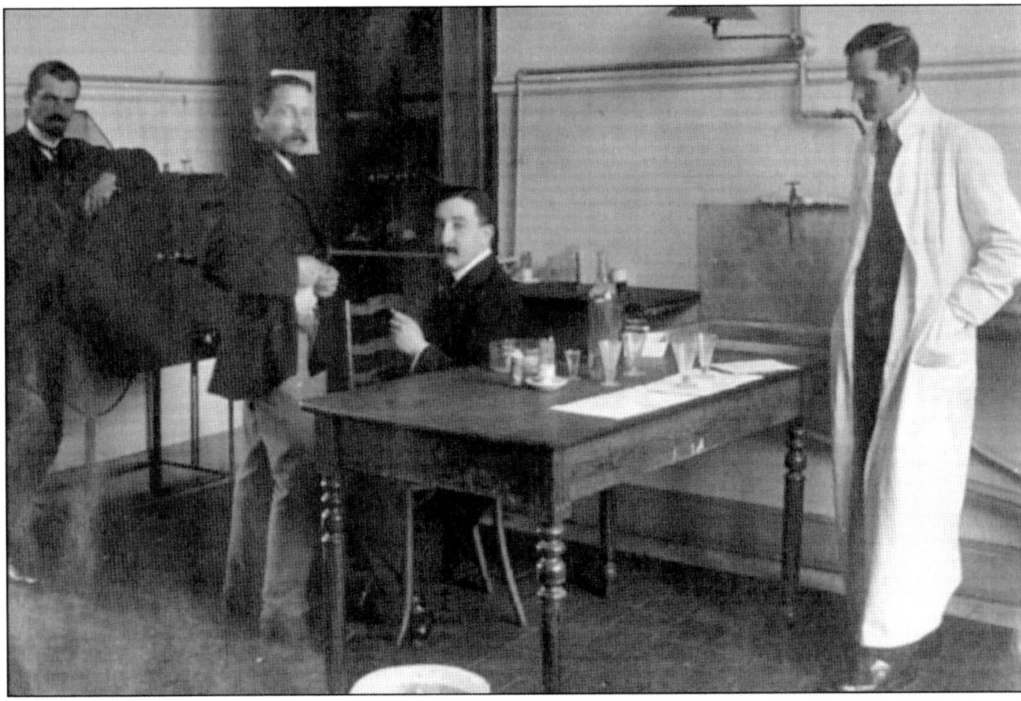

Canadian pathologist John Gerald Fitzgerald spent a year at Danvers State Hospital continuing to build the pathology library. Originally from Toronto, Fitzgerald was fascinated with bacteriology and the work of Louis Pasteur and Robert Koch. He came to Harvard on a research grant and set out to find whether or not certain forms of madness might be caused by infection. Eventually, Fitzgerald himself would succumb to major depression, attempting suicide a number of times. After being released from treatment at the Hartford Retreat, Fitzgerald was again hospitalized for an attempted overdose. While in the hospital, he took a knife and cut his femoral artery, causing him to bleed out. (Above John Gray; below, Kim Albright.)

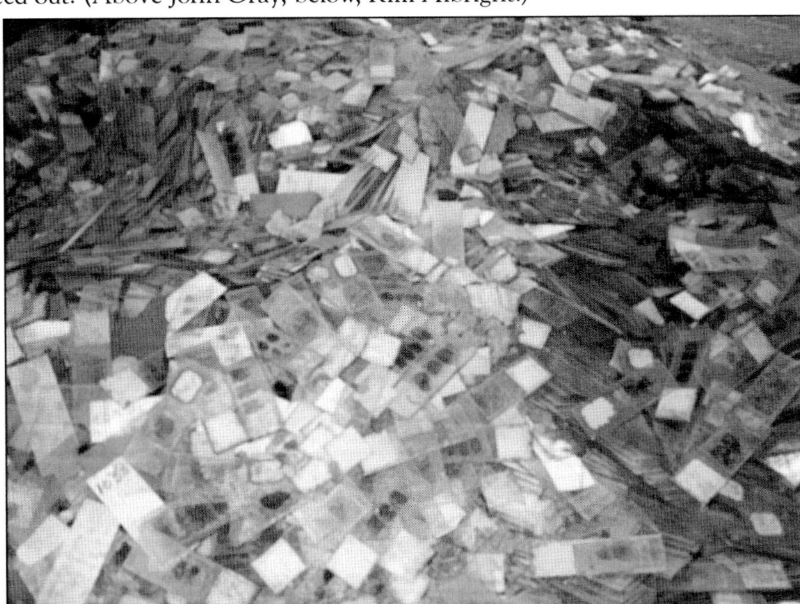

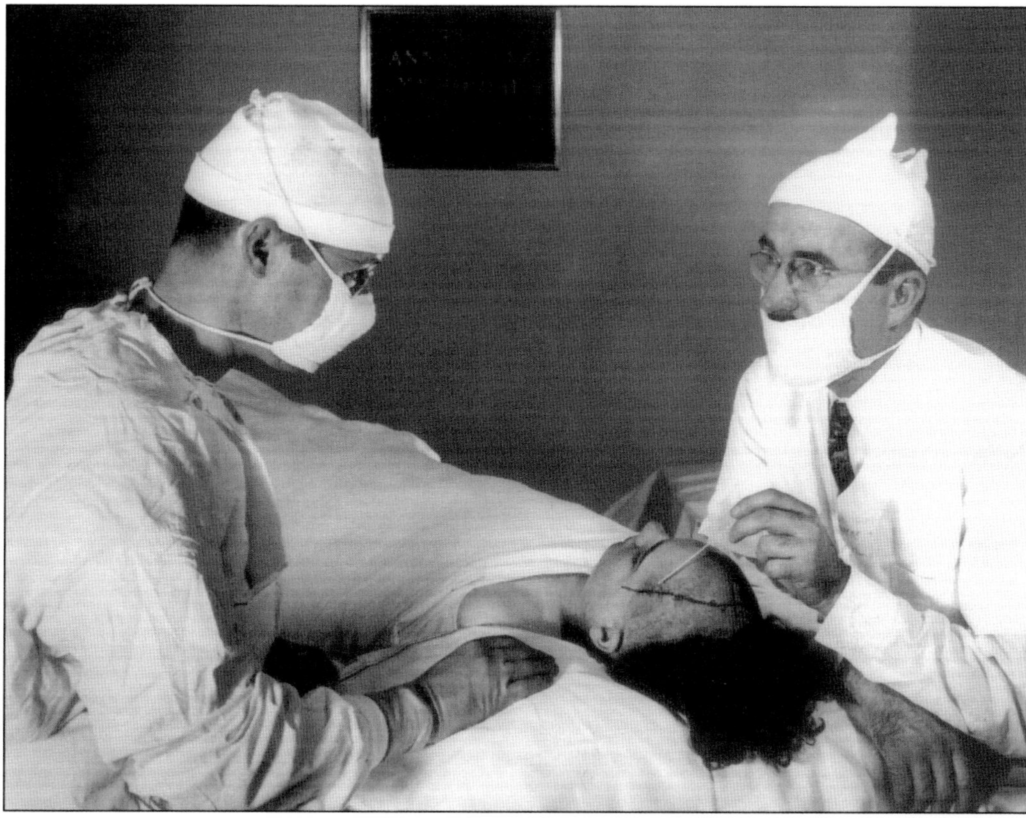

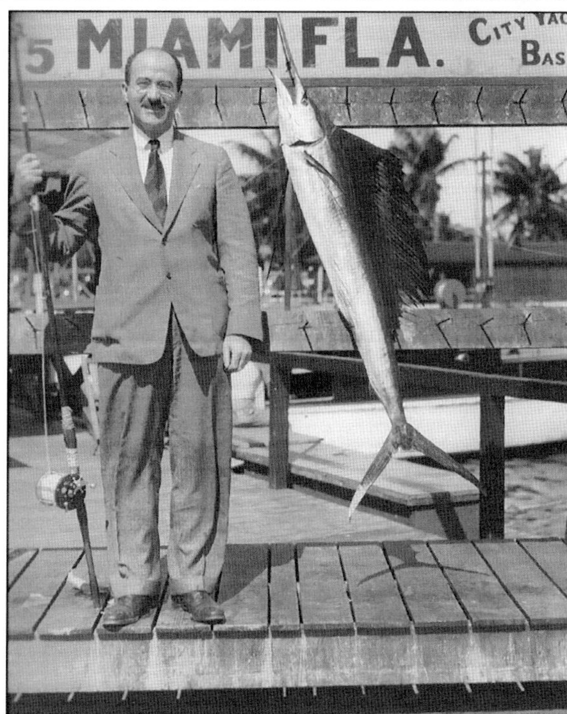

Walter Freeman was an American neurologist best known for perfecting the process of the prefrontal lobotomy. The procedure was performed by inserting an ice pick through the orbital socket and destroying nerve tissue in the frontal lobe of the brain. This limited the emotional responses in the patient and controlled the symptoms of mental illness. Dr. Freeman performed hundreds of lobotomies at Danvers State Hospital, earning it the nickname "the Birthplace of the Lobotomy." Freeman performed an estimated 3,500 lobotomies. He famously lobotomized Rosemary Kennedy in 1914, leaving her incontinent and unable to speak. (Both, Jack El-Hai.)

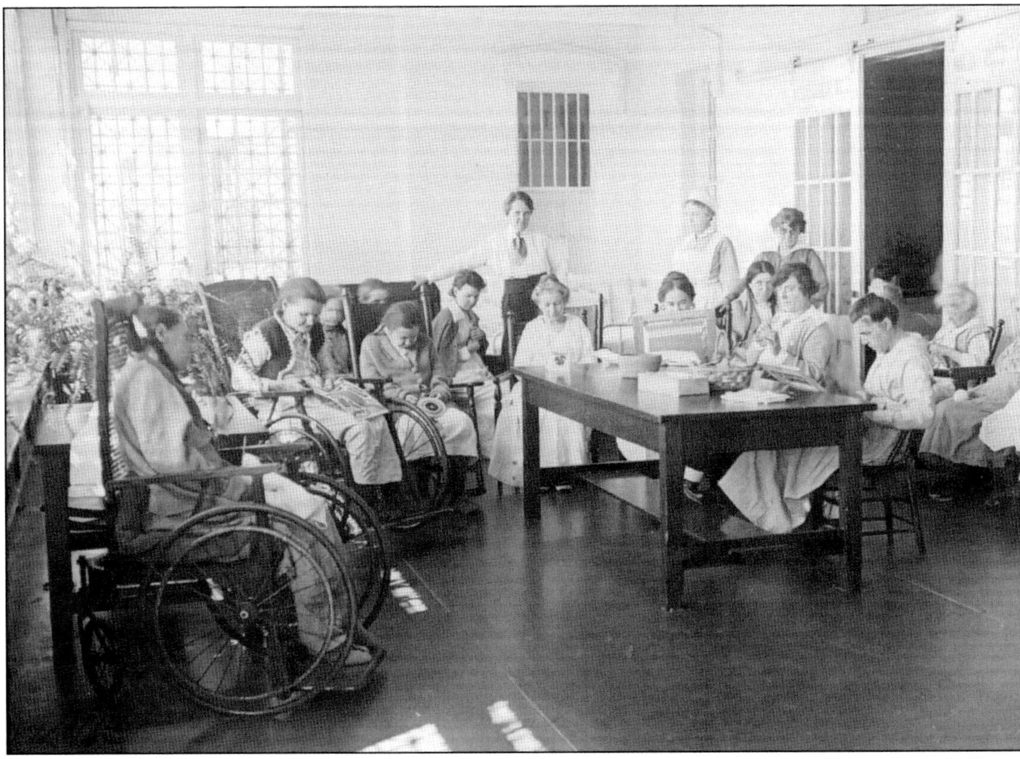

As part of its progressive approach to moral treatment and the eventual "cure" for mental illness, Danvers State Hospital began making use of occupational therapy early on. Patients engaged in a number of daily activities ranging from crafting shoes and stuffing mattresses to making small repairs to the buildings and grounds. Patient labor was used to dig tunnels and pour foundations, as well as on the farm and in the gardens. At one time, nearly 40 percent of the patient population worked on the farm. Occupational therapy groups such as those pictured were often run by patients. (Both, Ben Kenny.)

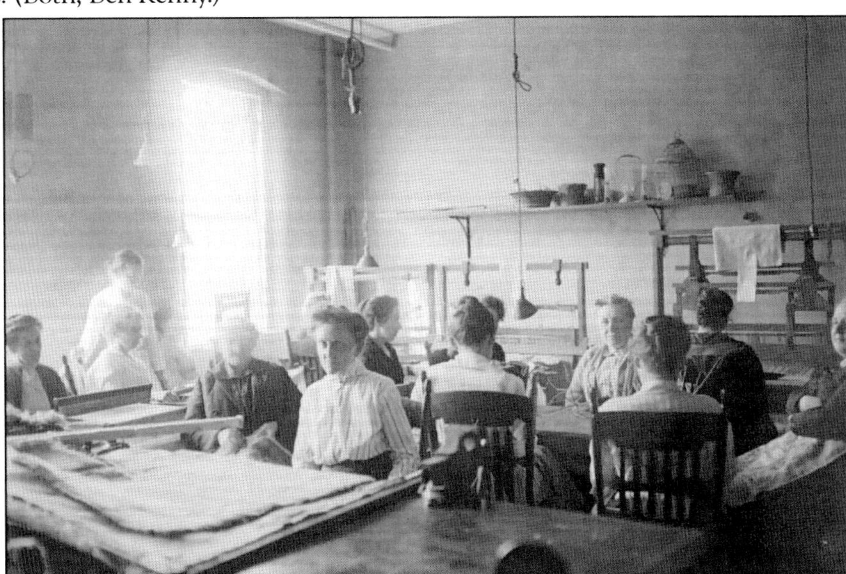

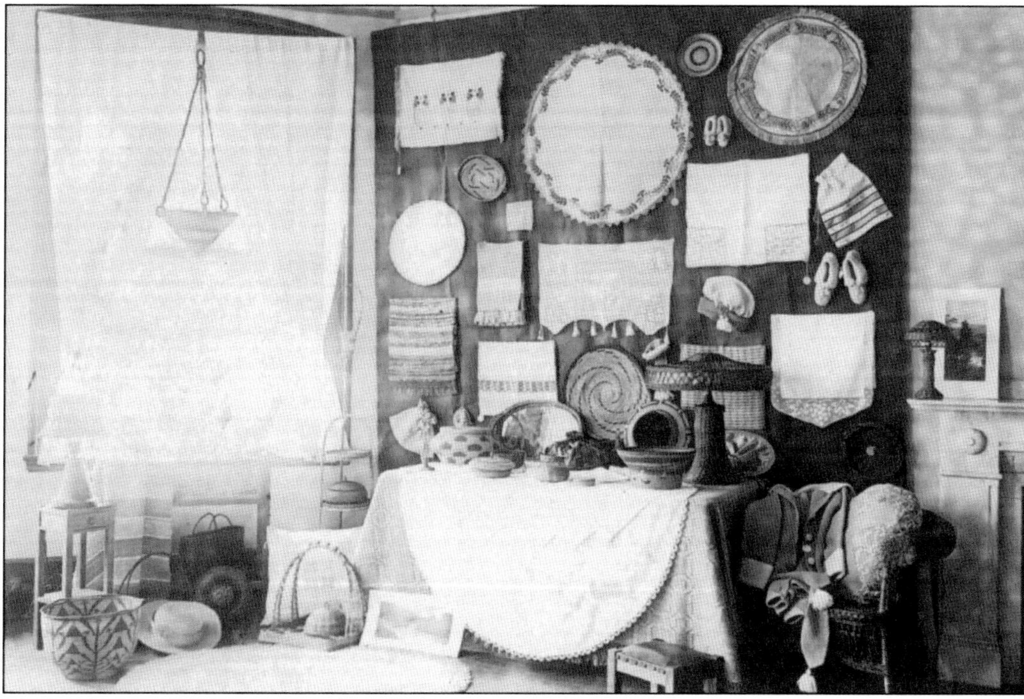

Under the watchful eye of ward staff, the patients wove textiles and practiced basic life skills by completing kindergarten-level readiness activities. Patient occupational therapy groups also made woven baskets, needlepoint pillows, booties, and clothing. The patient-made crafts were exhibited at the Boston Mechanics Hall Textile Show in 1916 and again at Stoneham in 1919. The items were displayed along with information about the hospital's latest therapeutic techniques, and some were even made available for purchase. In later years, Danvers would serve as a site for numerous occupational therapy internships. (Above, Ben Kenny; below, John Gray.)

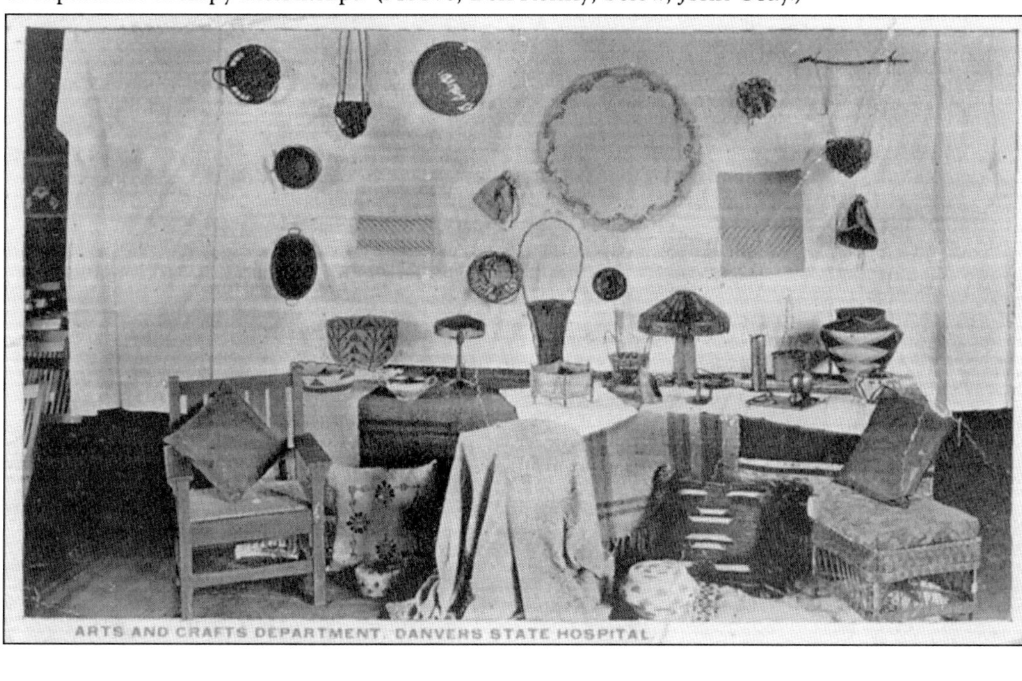

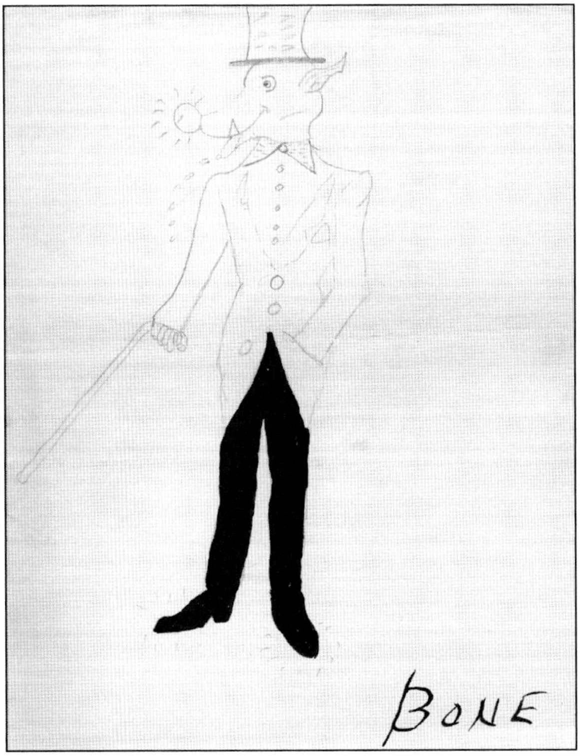

Art therapy was also a staple at Danvers State Hospital and remained so until it closed. Patients were generally encouraged to participate in psychotherapy, both individually and in groups, through creating individual artwork, such as these two drawings from the 1950s. Art was also used as yet another facet of occupational therapy, as it strengthens motor skills. In addition to drawing things they were working on in therapy, the patients often sketched and painted the asylum itself. Many of those paintings were then given to favorite staff members as gifts. Often, those drawings or paintings are all that are left of an individual patient and have remained treasured keepsakes for former staff members. (Both, John Archer.)

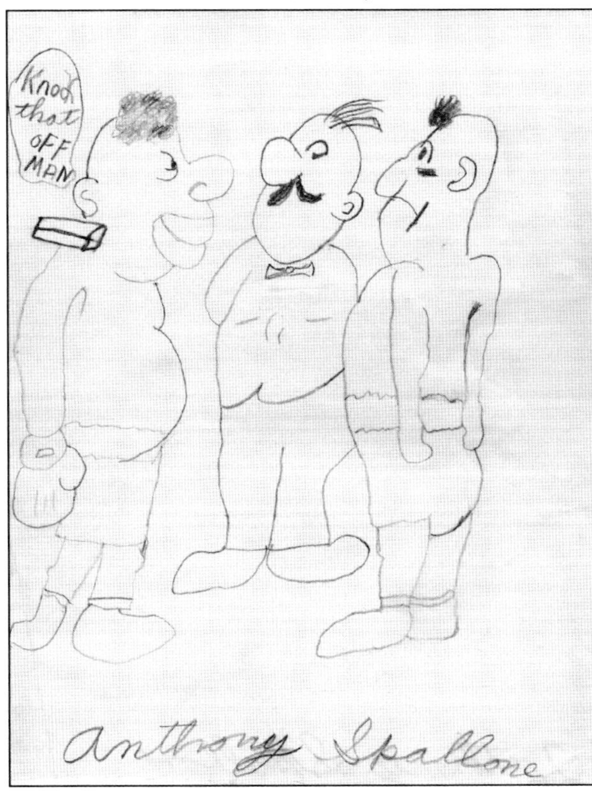

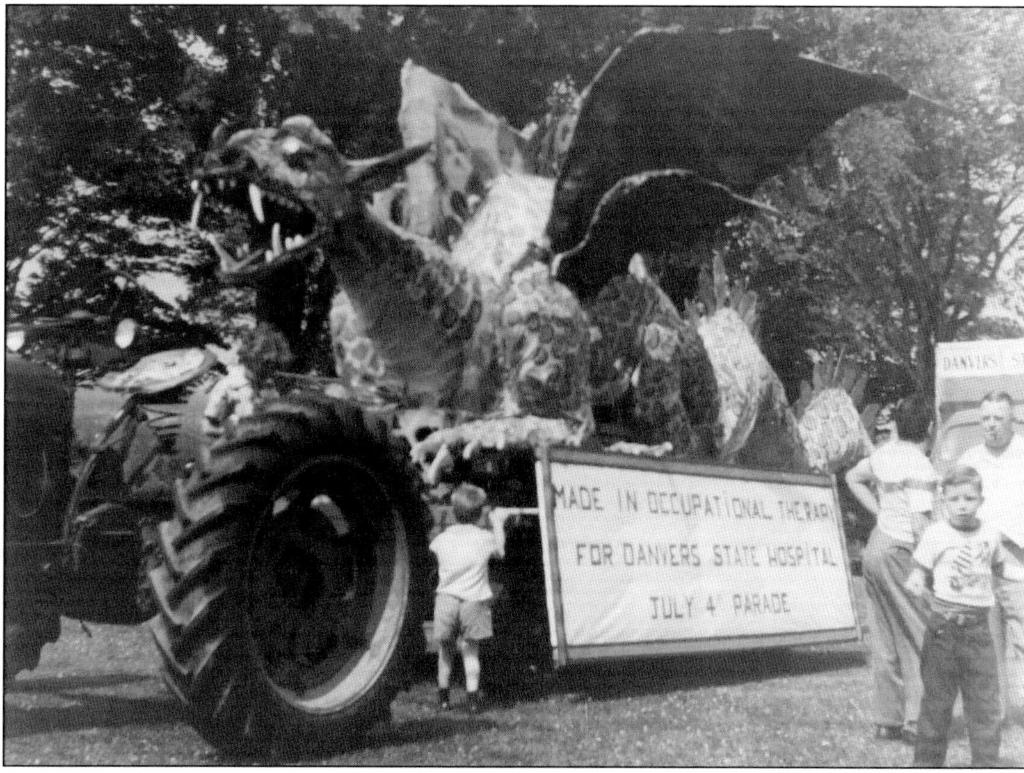

As early as the 1940s, artists and art educators began facilitating open studio classes for asylum patients. Group art therapy allowed for a break from traditional treatments by encouraging patients to also practice social skills and teamwork. The projects promoted communication and personal expression that allowed patients to bridge their inner and outer worlds. Pictured here is a life-sized papier-mâché dragon created by the patients in their occupational therapy group and turned into a float for a Fourth of July parade held sometime in the early 1950s. The celebration of holidays on the state hospital campus often featured decorations crafted by the patients. (Both, Massachusetts Archives.)

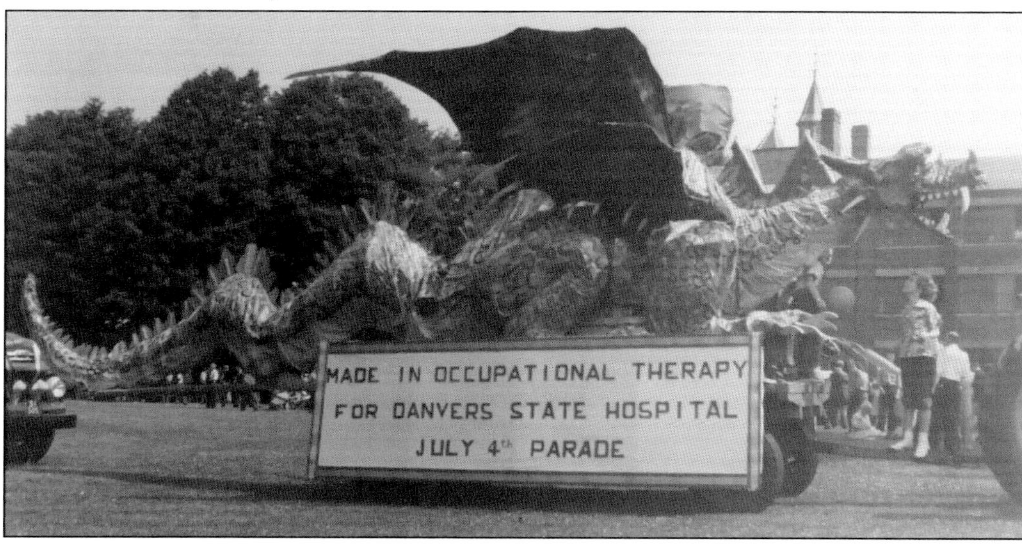

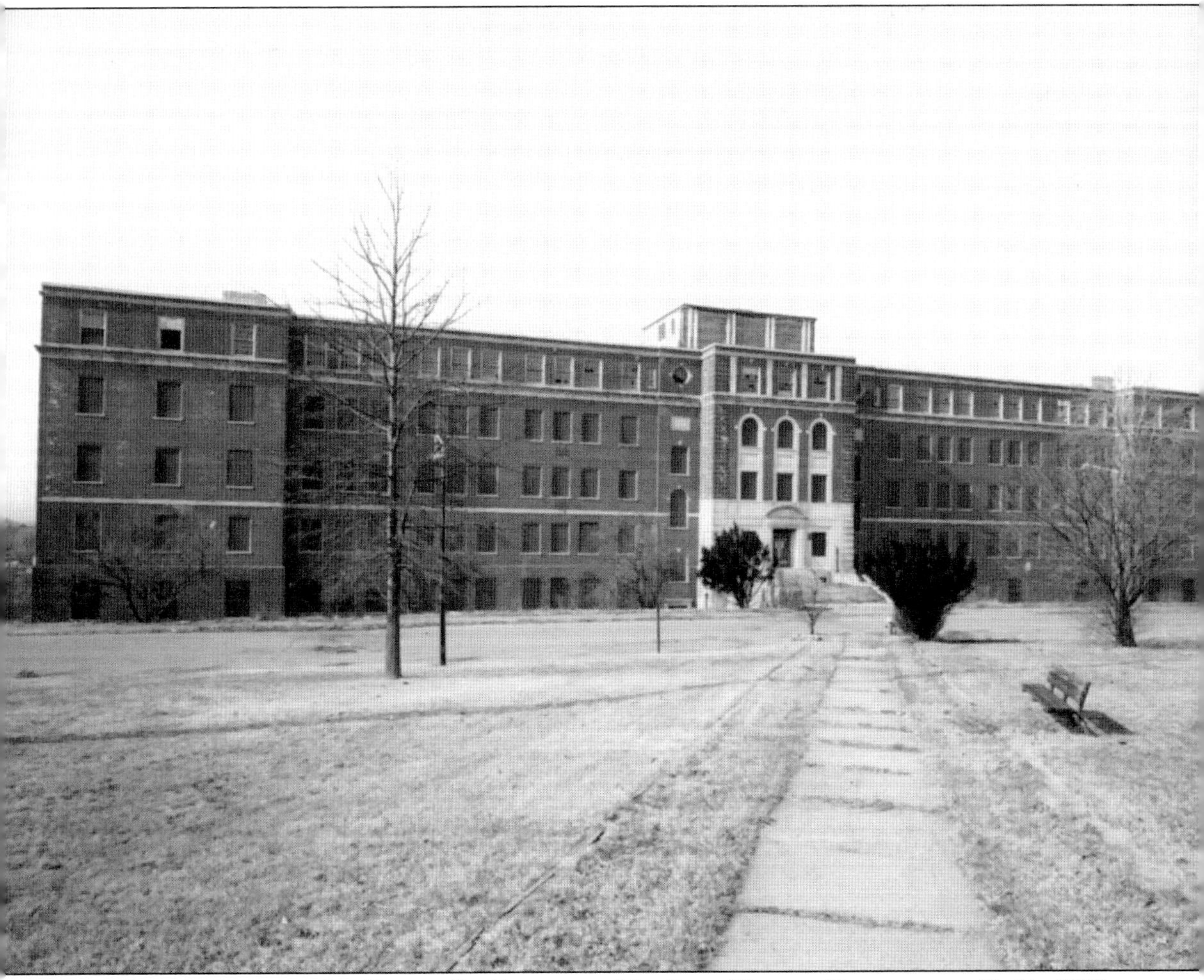

The 100,000-square-foot Bonner Building, named for Supt. Clarence Bonner, was added in 1955 as a general medical facility, but eventually, all services were moved to Bonner as the main Kirkbride was being closed down. Former staffer Sharon Cook recalls a mural of *The Wizard of Oz*'s Yellow Brick Road painted by patients and profiled in the Department of Mental Health's newspaper. In 1966, a legal act allowed for the creation of a school for "mentally retarded" children on the Danvers State Hospital campus to be called Hathorne State School. At that time, there were already four state schools for the feebleminded and developmentally disabled open and operating in Massachusetts. The Hathorne State School would eventually become the Hogan Regional Center and remains in operation. (Danvers Archival Center, Danvers, Massachusetts.)

Three

LIFE AT DANVERS

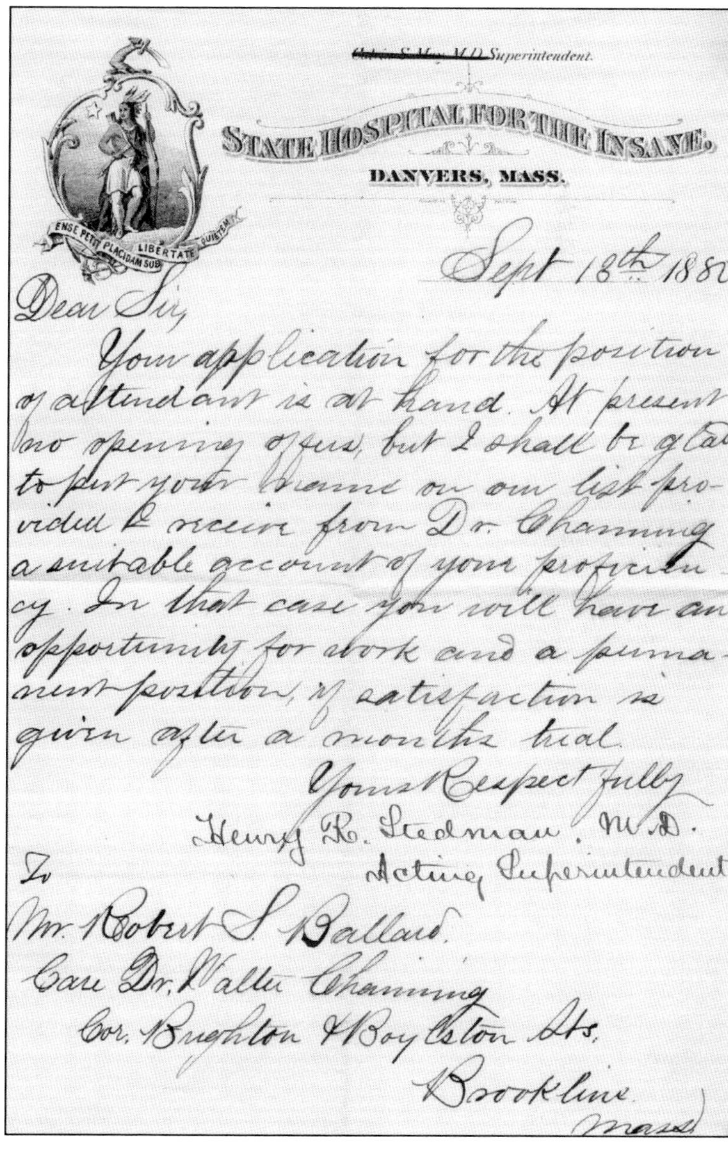
M.D. Superintendent.

STATE HOSPITAL FOR THE INSANE.

DANVERS, MASS.

ENSE PETIT PLACIDAM SUB LIBERTATE QUIETEM

Sept 18th 1880

Dear Sir,

Your application for the position of attendant is at hand. At present no opening offers, but I shall be glad to put your name on our list provided I receive from Dr. Channing a suitable account of your proficiency. In that case you will have an opportunity for work and a permanent position, if satisfaction is given after a months trial.

Yours Respectfully

Henry R. Stedman. M.D.

Acting Superintendent

To

Mr. Robert S. Ballard.

Care Dr. Walter Channing

Cor. Brighton & Boylston Sts.

Brookline.

Mass.

Even before the asylum opened its doors, employment at Danvers Lunatic Hospital was highly sought after. Male attendants in 1901 made on average anywhere between $20 and $37 per month, while female attendants averaged between $15 and $30 monthly. Outside of the asylum, the average monthly salary was a mere $10. Pictured here is a letter from acting superintendent Henry Stedman confirming receipt of a request for a job as an attendant in 1880. (Jett Chapman.)

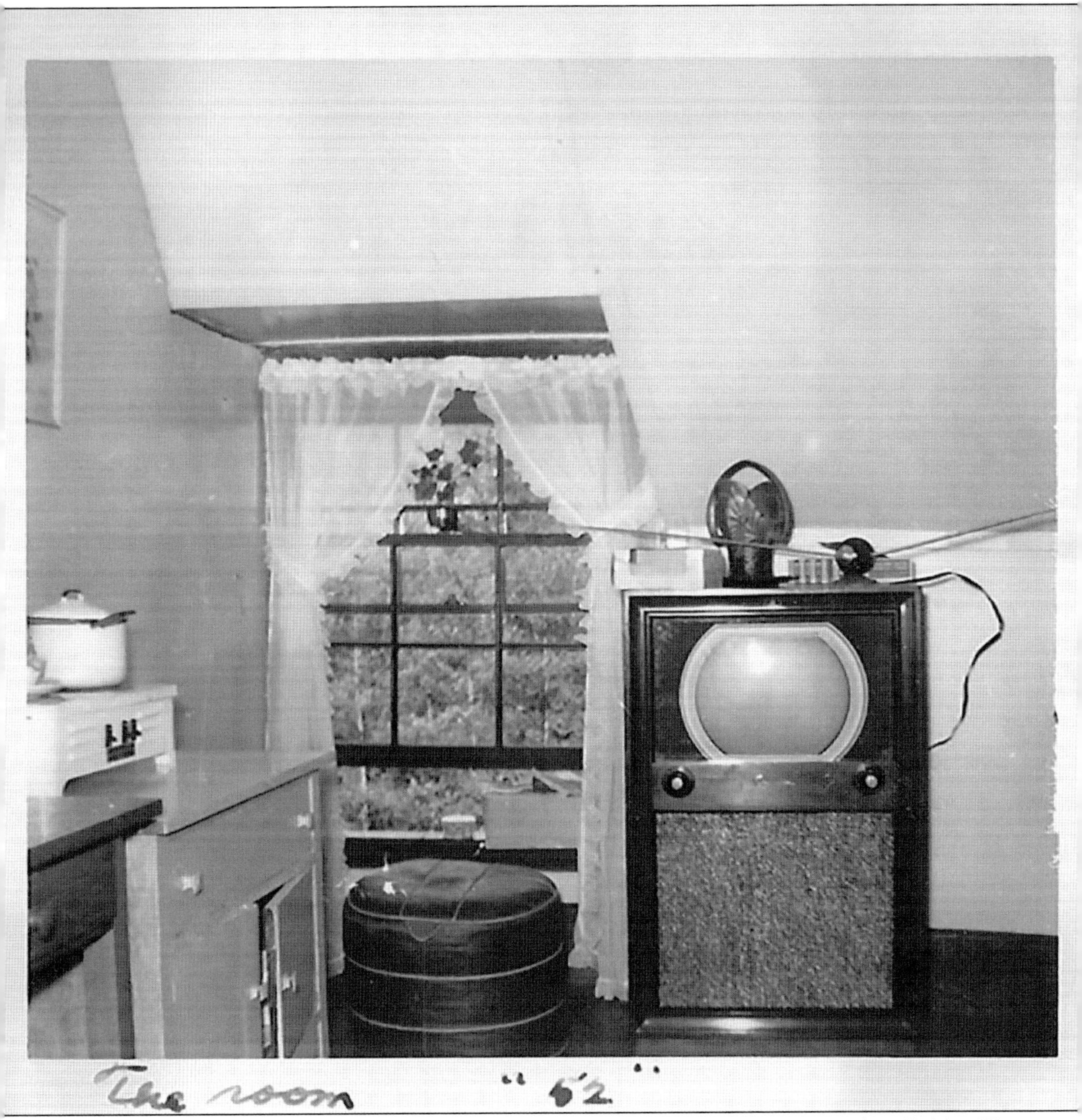

Working at Danvers State Hospital created a family atmosphere for patients and staff alike. The nurses' houses were staffed by house mothers, with the nurses living dorm style, sharing common living spaces while making their rooms their own. Pictured here is a room belonging to Alberta, a nurse on the wards through the 1950s who documented her time at Danvers in a large collection of photographs. Well into the later years of the hospital's operations, the staff continued to live on campus, as did the superintendent and his assistant. By the late 1960s, staff were even living in studio apartments in the upper floors of the Kirkbride. (John Gray.)

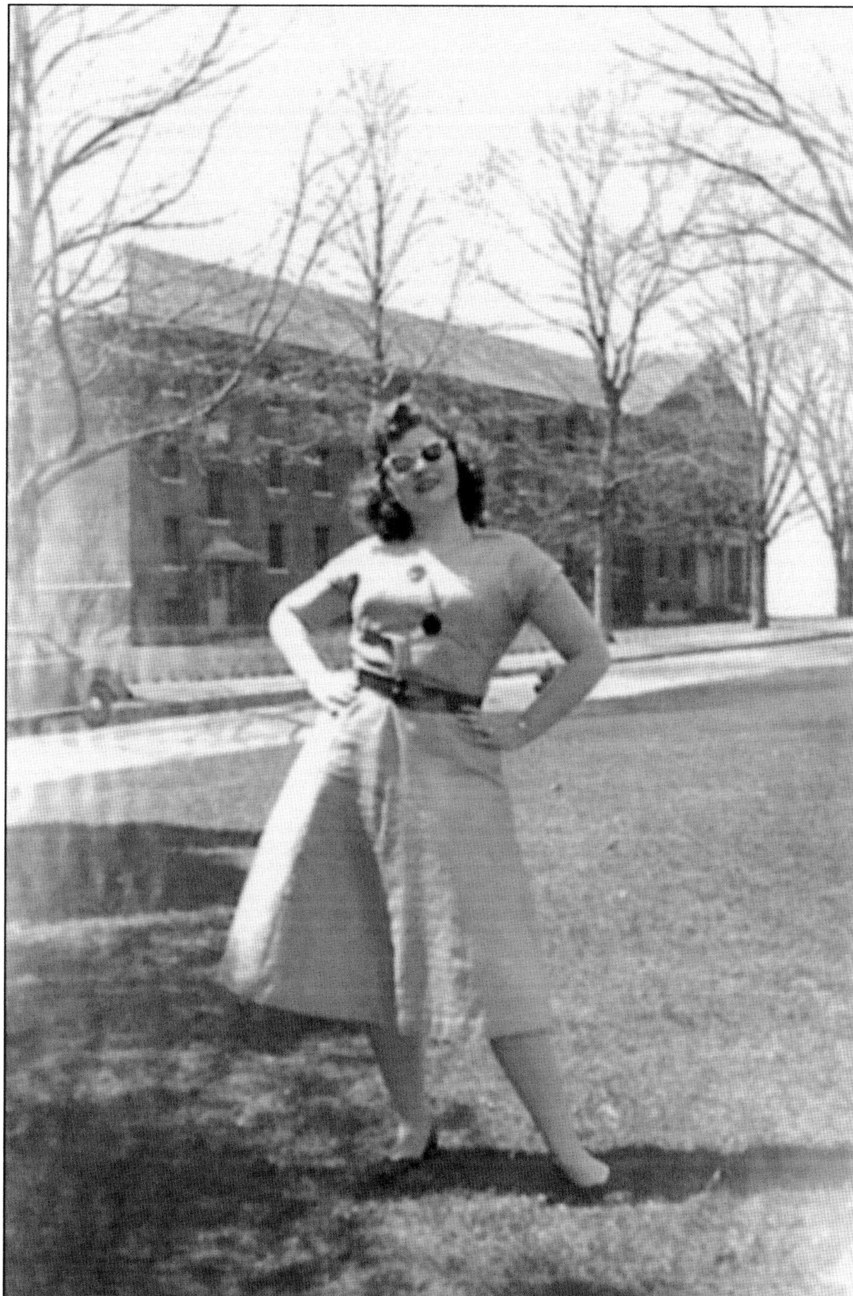

In the first year of its operation, the state hospital employed approximately 73 of a total 305 patients (139 males and 166 females), and most of them were diagnosed with either acute or chronic mania. In the first superintendent's report after receiving the hospital from the state, Calvin May boasted that all of those patients were maintained on two unlocked wards. By 1898, the State Board of Insanity considered Danvers a leader in the implementation of progressive and humanitarian tenets, one of the "most advanced institutions of the kind in the country providing all practical means possible for the intelligent treatment of insanity as a disease" by emphasizing mental hygiene and calling for the professional training of all hospital staff. (John Gray.)

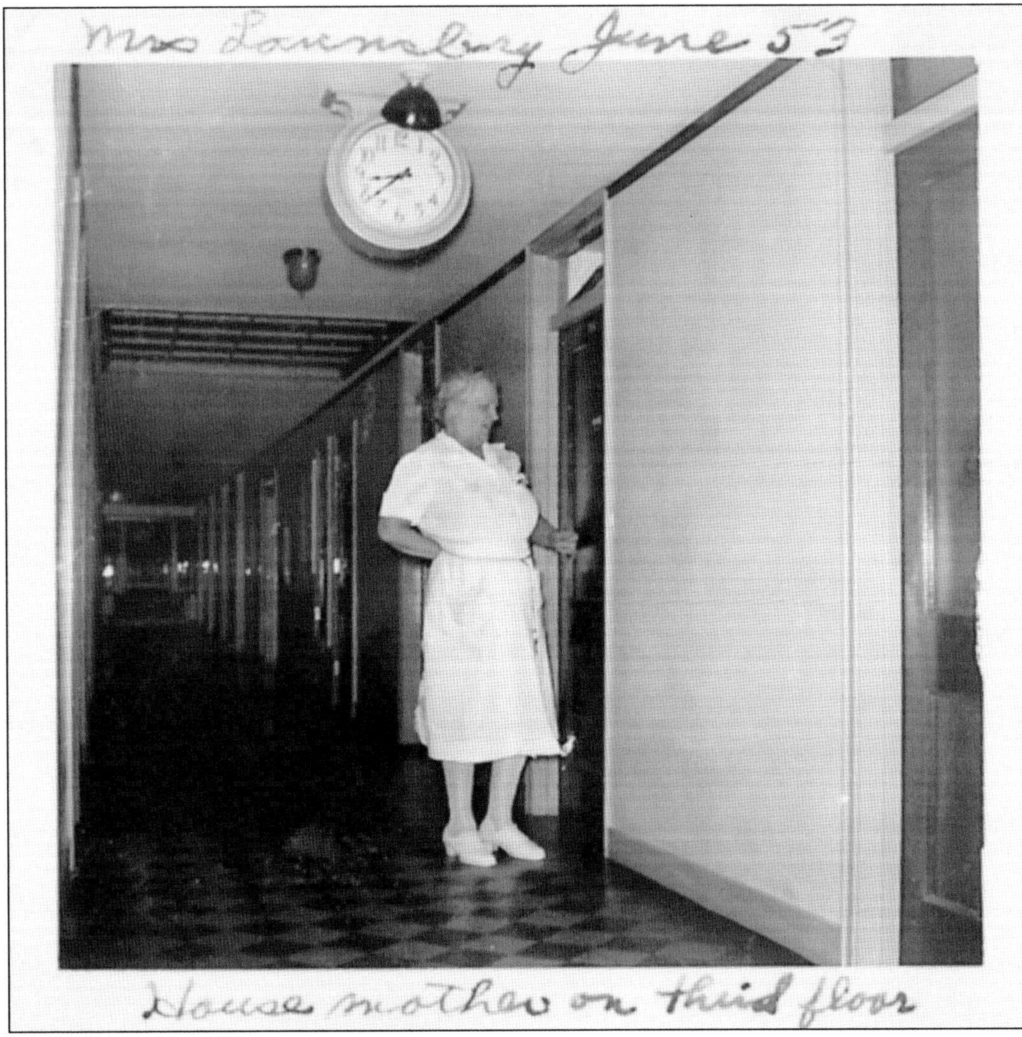

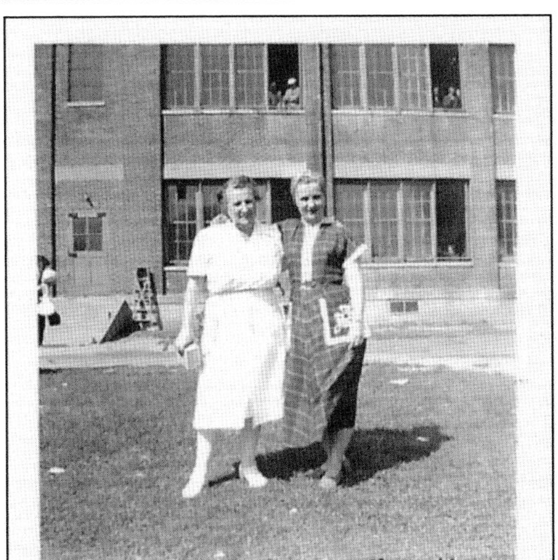

The nurses were supervised by a house mother though in some cases the nurses employed on the wards worked side by side with their own mothers (as in the photograph at left). Often, generations of family worked at the state hospital, some couples meeting at the asylum and later marrying. Children were born and raised on the campuses of state hospitals nationwide. In later years, married couples were housed in Gray Gables, which originally served as a nurses' dorm. Around that same time, Farm Hall was reserved for hired staff, while patients were moved to Grove Hall, a step-up living arrangement that was an earned privilege. (Both, Karen Bourdelais.)

Despite its cutting-edge treatment of the mentally ill, the asylum did not have full general medical facilities for employees. Shown here is a bill for an ambulance ride taken by nurse Hazel Fisher from Gray Gables to Salem Hospital; it was approved for payment by Dr. Peter Hagopian. (David Walsh.)

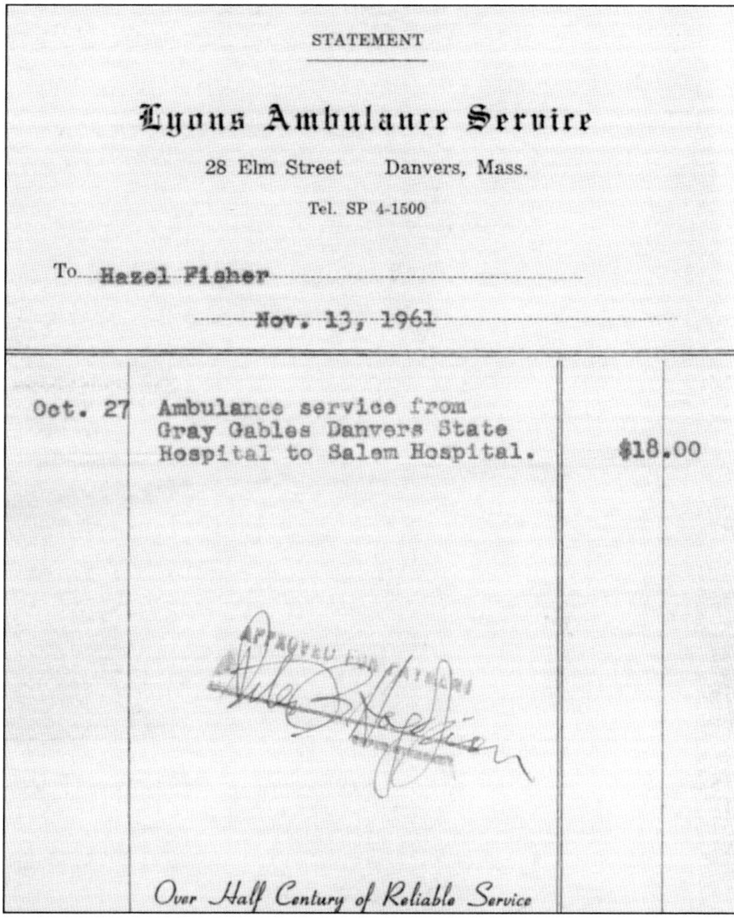

STATEMENT

Lyons Ambulance Service

28 Elm Street Danvers, Mass.

Tel. SP 4-1500

To Hazel Fisher

Nov. 13, 1961

Oct. 27	Ambulance service from Gray Gables Danvers State Hospital to Salem Hospital.	$18.00

Over Half Century of Reliable Service

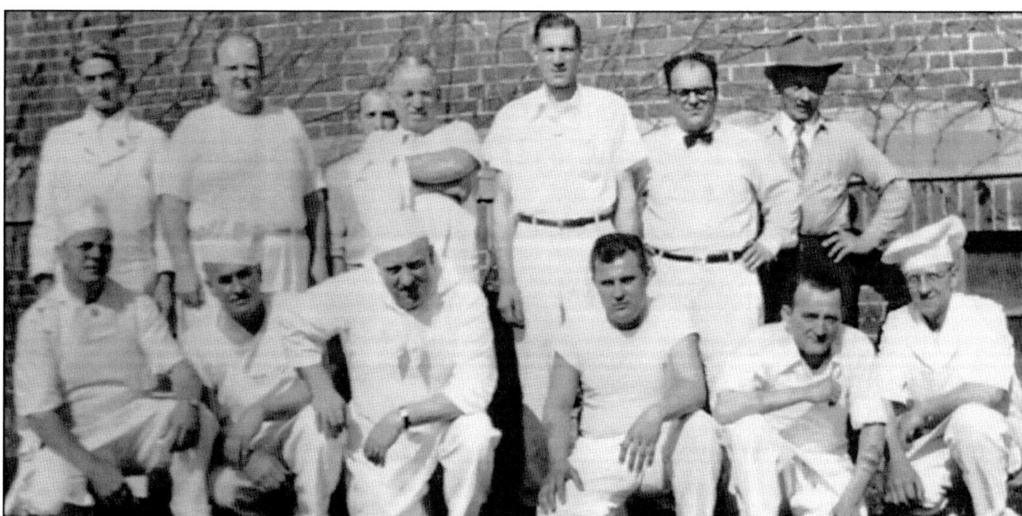

A team of cooks turned the meat and produce from the farm into meals for everyone living on campus at Danvers State Hospital. Milk was served regularly, a product of the state hospital's dairy herd. The farm provided the kitchen with beef, pork, and eggs as well. (John Gray.)

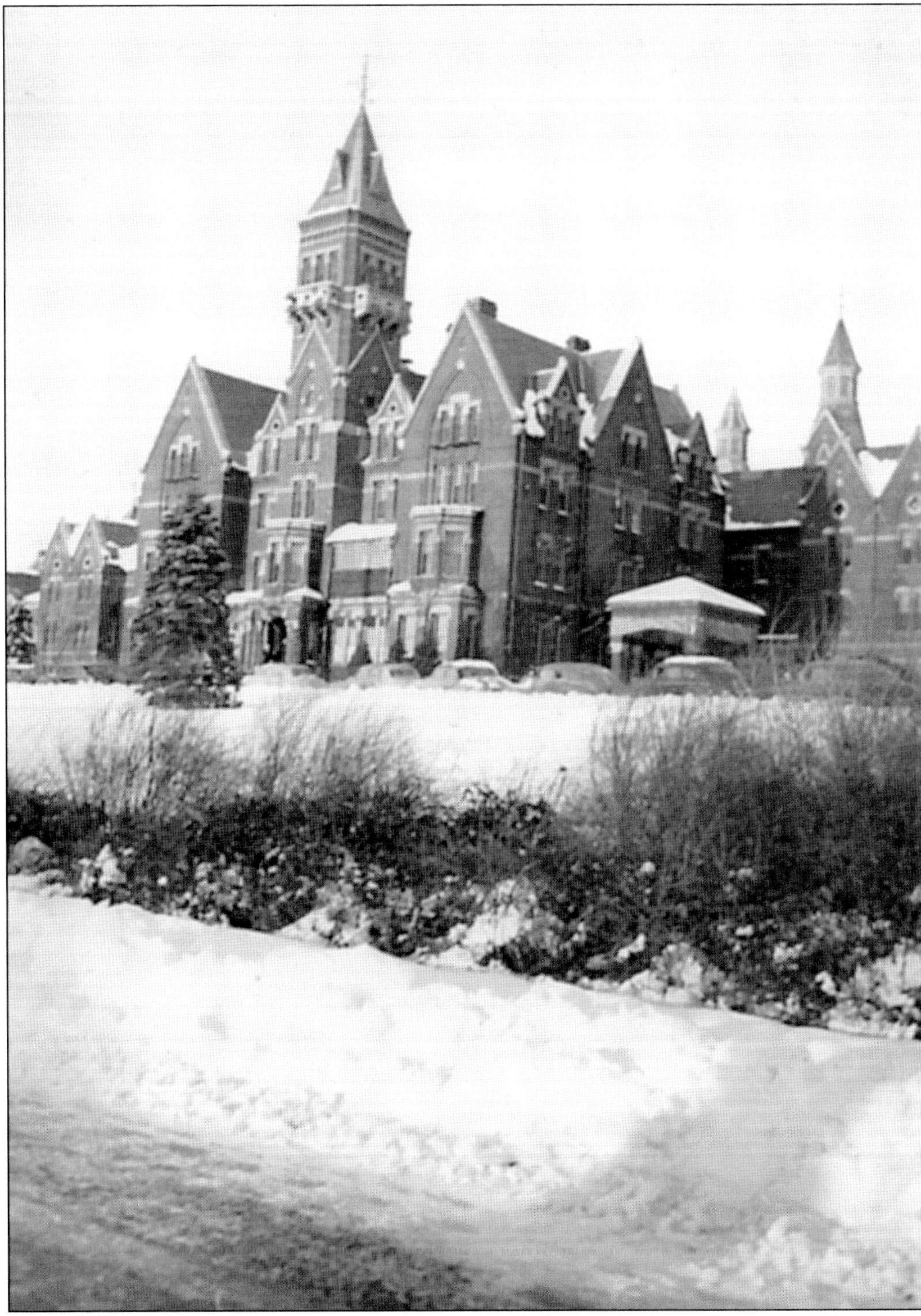

Pictured here is the main administrative building of the Kirkbride in the winter of 1952 and again in 1953. To the right of the main entrance is the porte cochere that was later demolished to make way for a stair tower. (John Gray.)

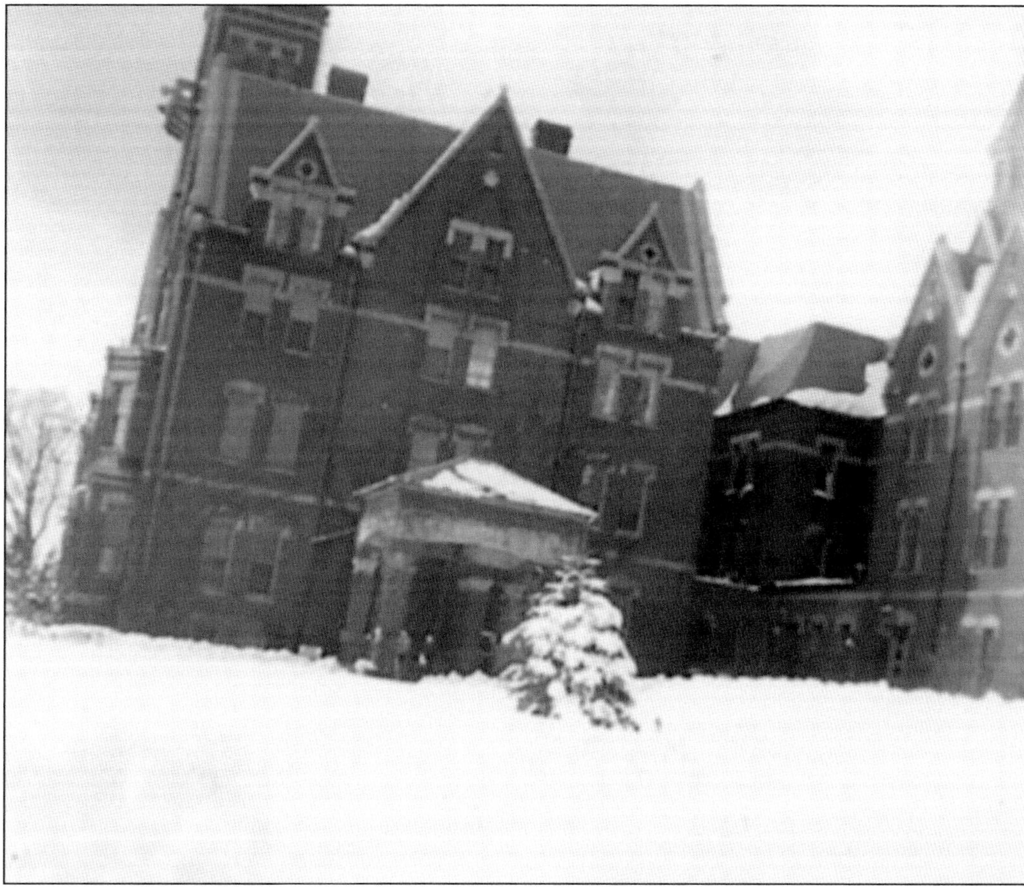

The windows on the ward sun porches are shuttered tight against the bitter cold of New England winter. In the event that patients needed to be transported to other buildings on campus, an extensive tunnel system connected the Kirkbride with its outbuildings. Both images were taken by Alberta, a nurse on the wards in the early 1950s. (John Gray.)

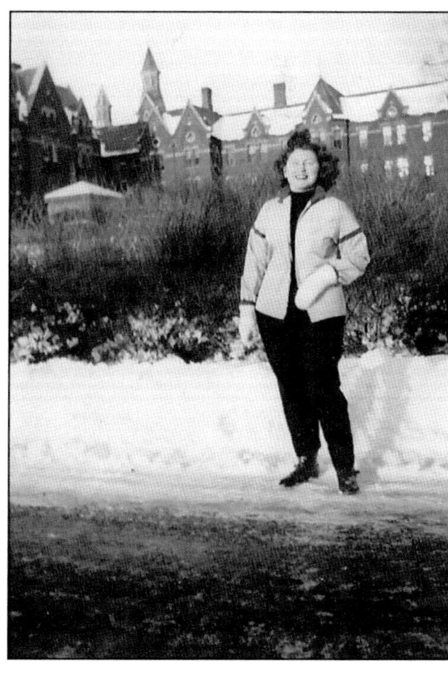

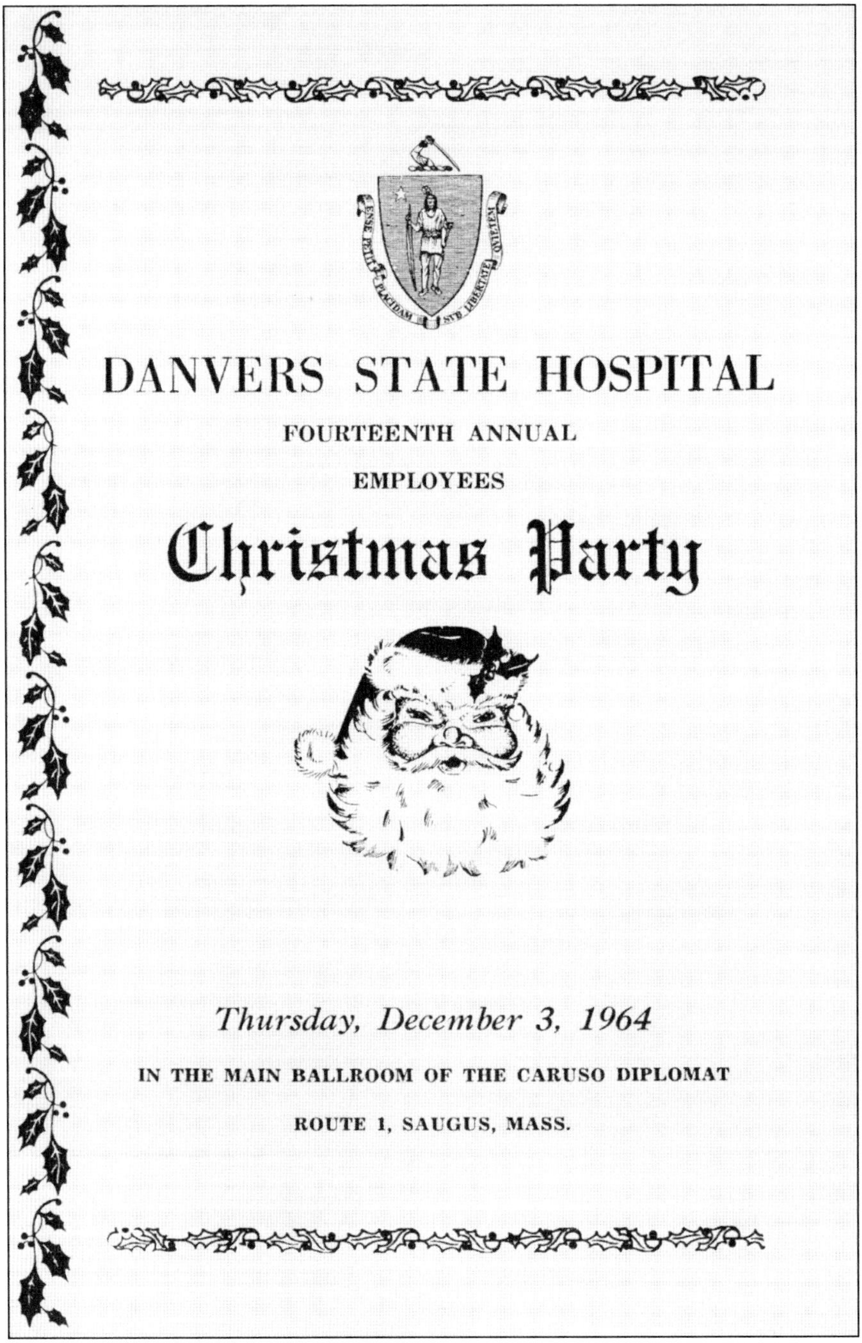

DANVERS STATE HOSPITAL

FOURTEENTH ANNUAL

EMPLOYEES

Christmas Party

Thursday, December 3, 1964

IN THE MAIN BALLROOM OF THE CARUSO DIPLOMAT

ROUTE 1, SAUGUS, MASS.

Pictured here is a flyer for an employee holiday party hosted at the Caruso Diplomat in Saugus (now demolished). Staff had the opportunity to attend with their families and celebrate separate from the patients. Patient holiday events were held at the hospital itself, with each ward having their own party of sorts. Many times, staff members would purchase gifts for the patients, especially those without family, as well as decorate the wards for the holidays with trees and streamers. Early annual reports also suggest that town residents made donations toward patient Christmas gifts. (Amanda Kohut.)

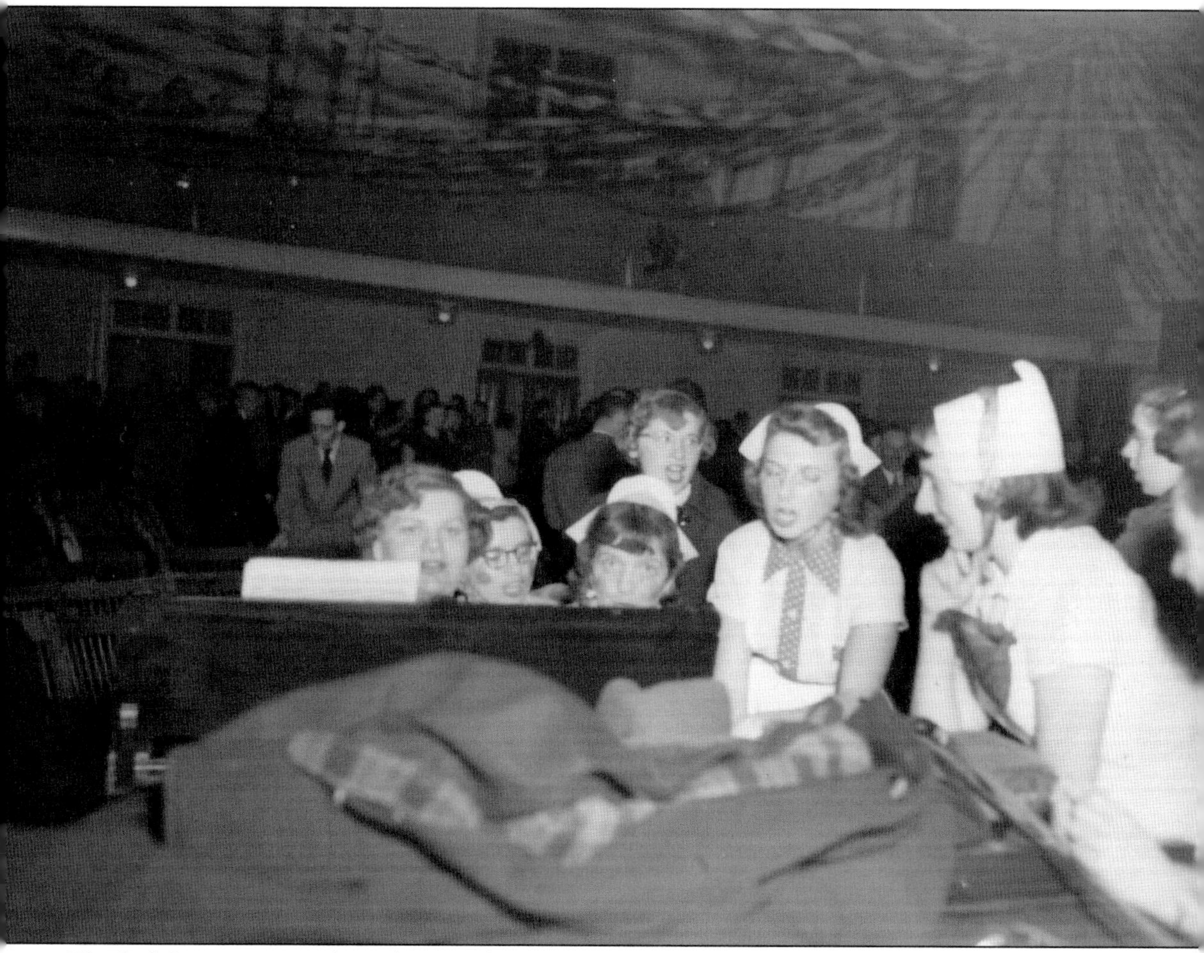

The holidays were not the only time that entertainment was provided, though Christmas was certainly the most elaborate. From the moment the hospital opened its doors, it was important that patients be provided with adequate opportunities to socialize and enjoy themselves. Weekly dances were recorded as early as 1880. The program of patient entertainment grew to include lectures on topics such as astronomy and Abraham Lincoln. Concerts were given by the Schubert Club from Boston as well as military bands. The 1888 annual report even lists a masquerade ball. Much of this entertainment was made possible by regular donations from townspeople and local businesses. (Karen Bourdelais.)

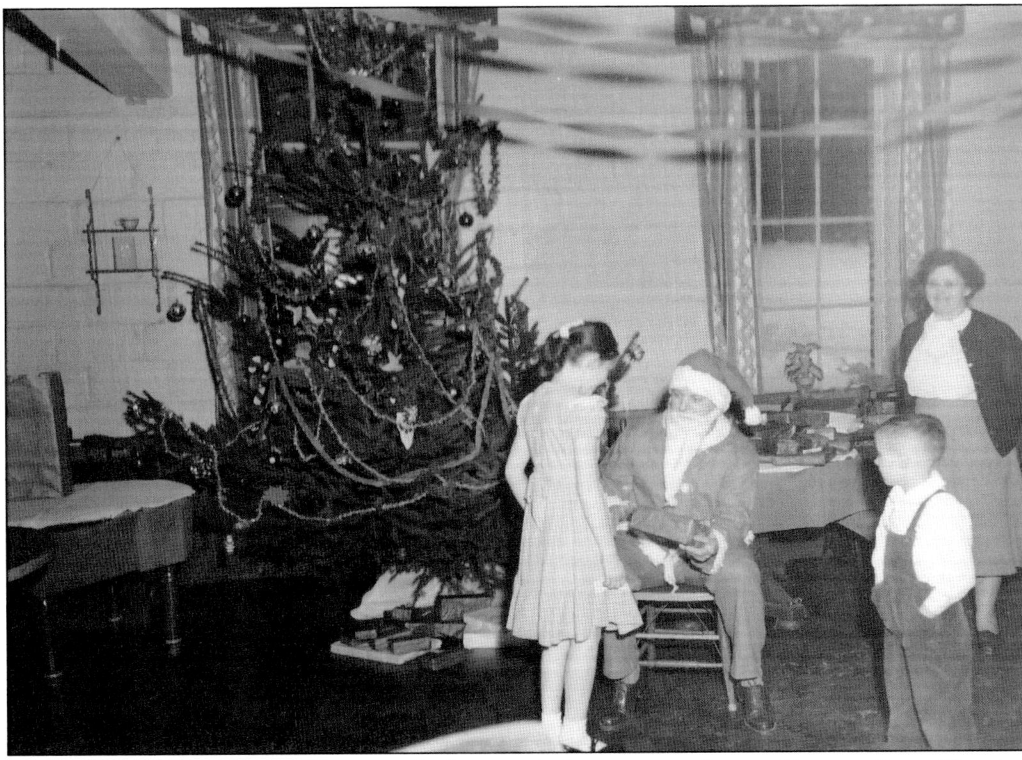

These images, found in a collection of ephemera belonging to a former Danvers State Hospital Auxiliary member, were likely taken at the 1964 Christmas party at the Caruso Diplomat. The remainder of the collection suggests that a small religious service was held as well along with an awards ceremony. Santa Claus would make an appearance and gifts were handed out to the children in attendance while their parents looked on. Tickets to the event were likely sold in advance, and the ballroom was decorated by hospital staff. Dr. Hagopian who served as superintendent that year was made honorary general chairman of the Christmas party committee. (Both, John Archer.)

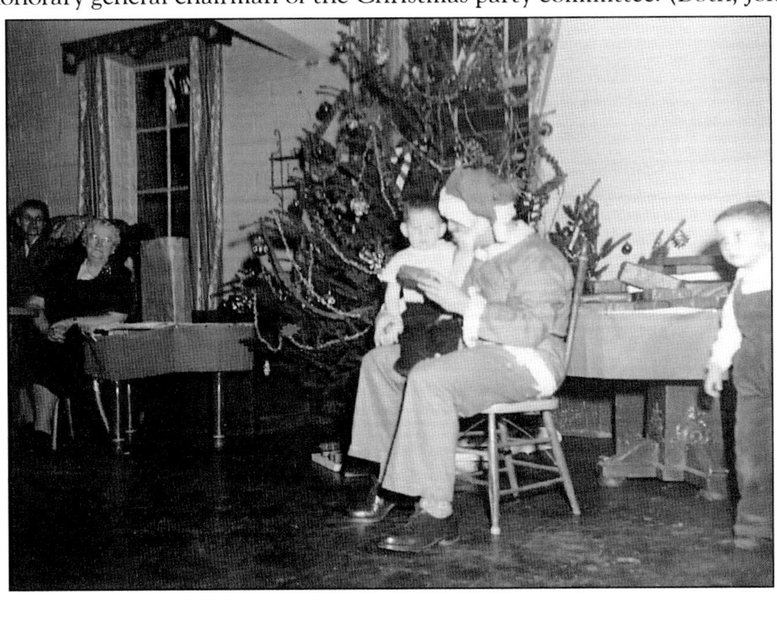

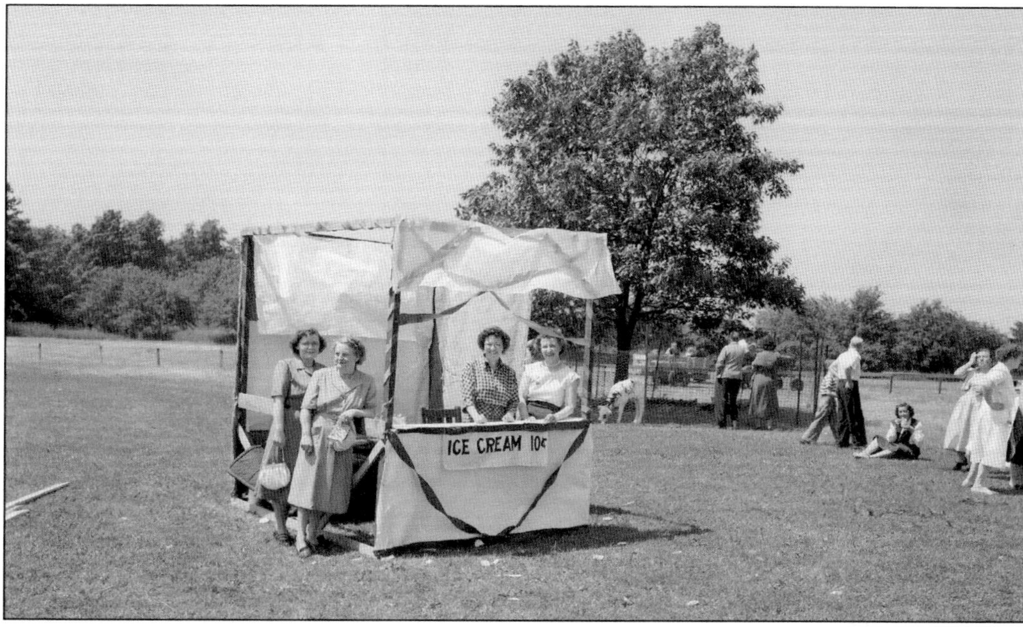

The Danvers State Hospital Auxiliary Committee hosted an annual country fair on the front lawn of the state hospital with livestock exhibitions, ice-cream stands, shows, and games. A number of booths were manned by hospital staff and community volunteers alike. Farm staff gave hay rides to the children, and others manned a hot dog stand inside the female summerhouse. The June 1955 fair was Davy Crockett themed, and announcements made by the committee promised members would be dressed in costume and that there would be a children's pet show. Music would be provided by a "hillbilly sextet." (Both, David Walsh.)

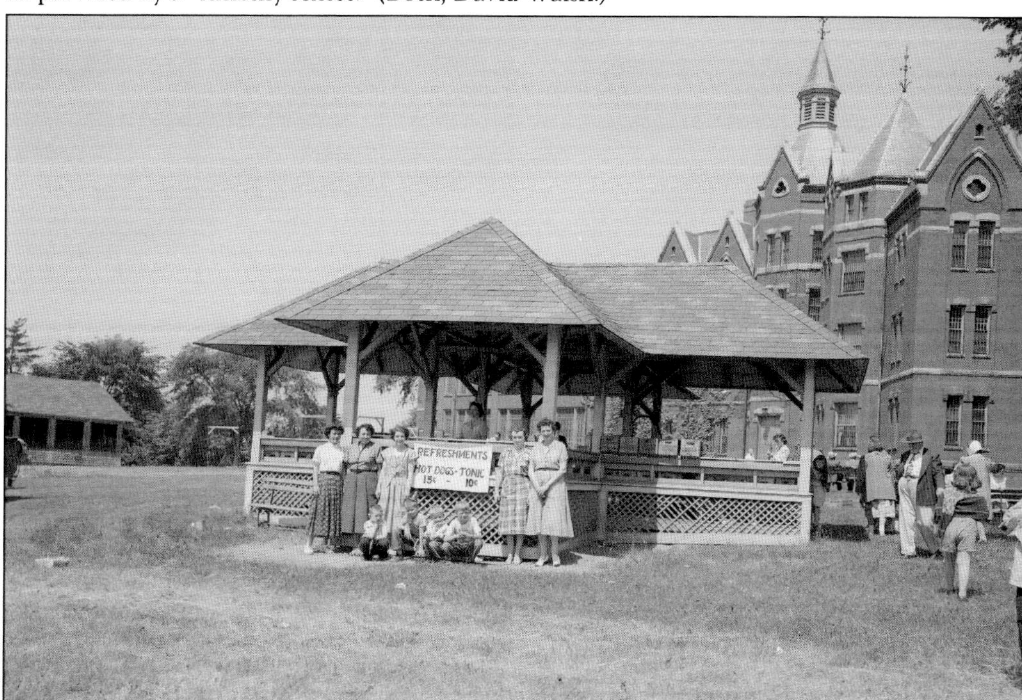

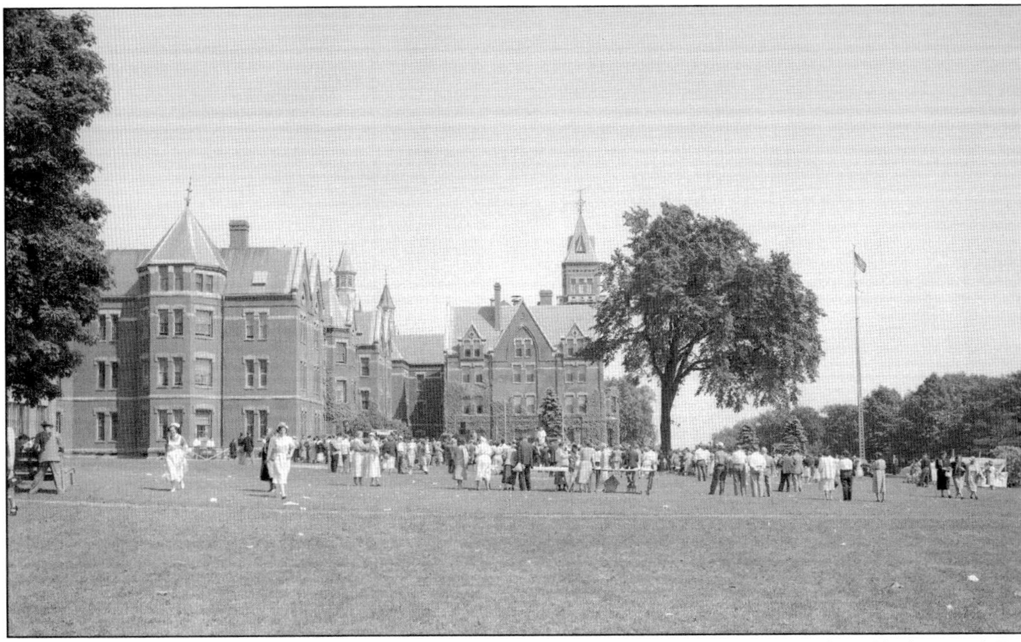

Children's games at Frontier Day included a penny toss, a sharpshooter booth called "Dead Eye Dick," and a Davey Crockett booth with staff members dressed up as famous Western characters such as Annie Oakley, Kit Carson, and Buffalo Bill. Along with the children's petting zoo, there was an activity called "rat race" that was filled with white rats. The event's announcement read, "Blaze a trail to the hospital grounds . . . and enjoy a few hours during Frontier Days at Danvers State Hospital," and the general public was invited. The event featured an auction sale of items donated by townspeople. (Both, David Walsh.)

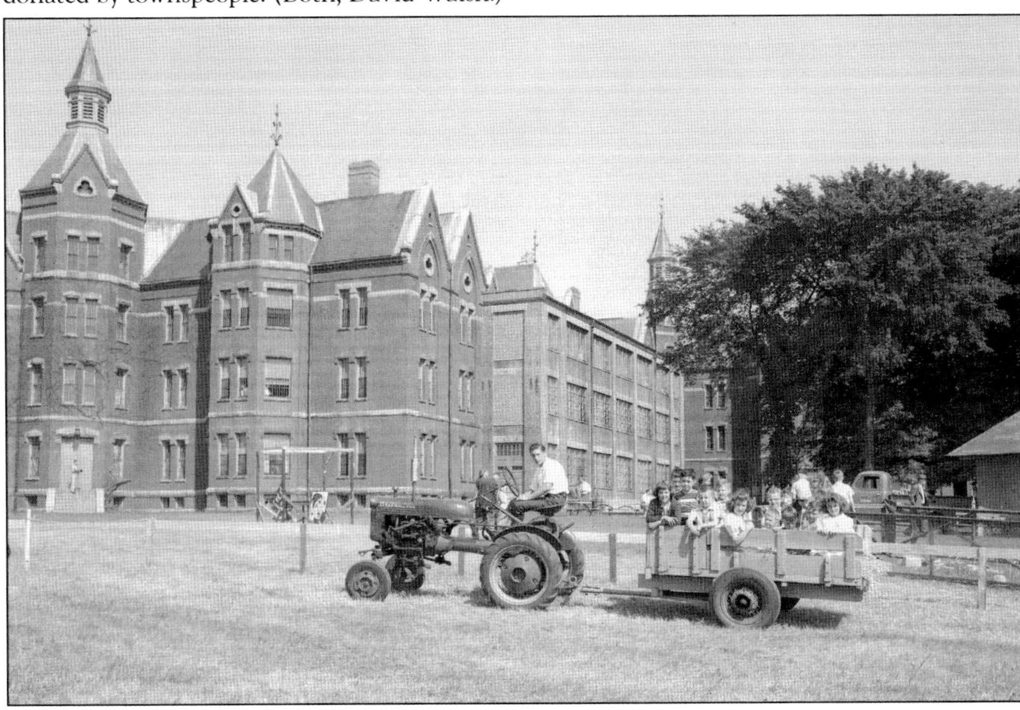

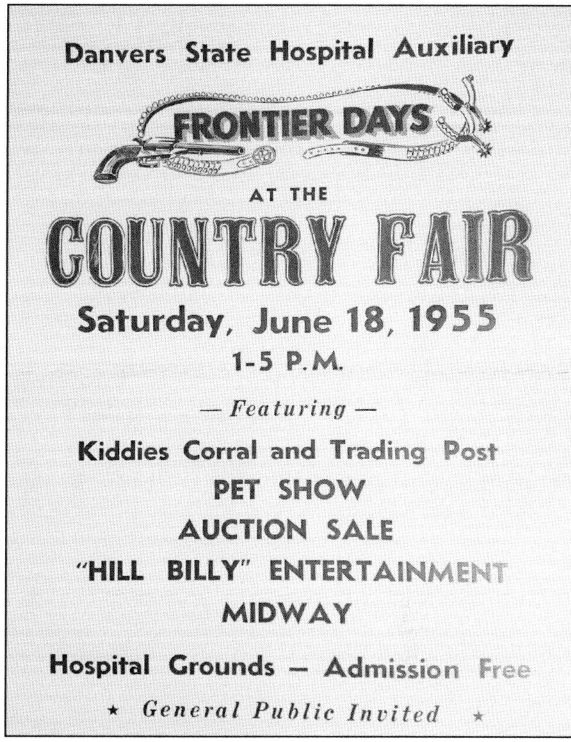
Danvers State Hospital Auxiliary
FRONTIER DAYS
AT THE
COUNTRY FAIR
Saturday, June 18, 1955
1-5 P.M.
— Featuring —
Kiddies Corral and Trading Post
PET SHOW
AUCTION SALE
"HILL BILLY" ENTERTAINMENT
MIDWAY
Hospital Grounds – Admission Free
★ General Public Invited ★

Family members and friends of both staff and patients were often invited to the state hospital for special events such as Frontier Day, pictured here on June 18, 1954. Frontier Day was a country fair complete with rides, games, and even a petting zoo. They held a parade and hosted a drum and bugle corps. Nurses and staff members manned drink stands and snack booths; stages for shows and platforms for guest speakers were constructed by the maintenance staff. There was a rolling canteen, handmade jewelry, and a booth featuring "needlework, novelties, and plants." Prizes raffled off included a picture, a pair of lamps, and a new chair. (Both, David Walsh.)

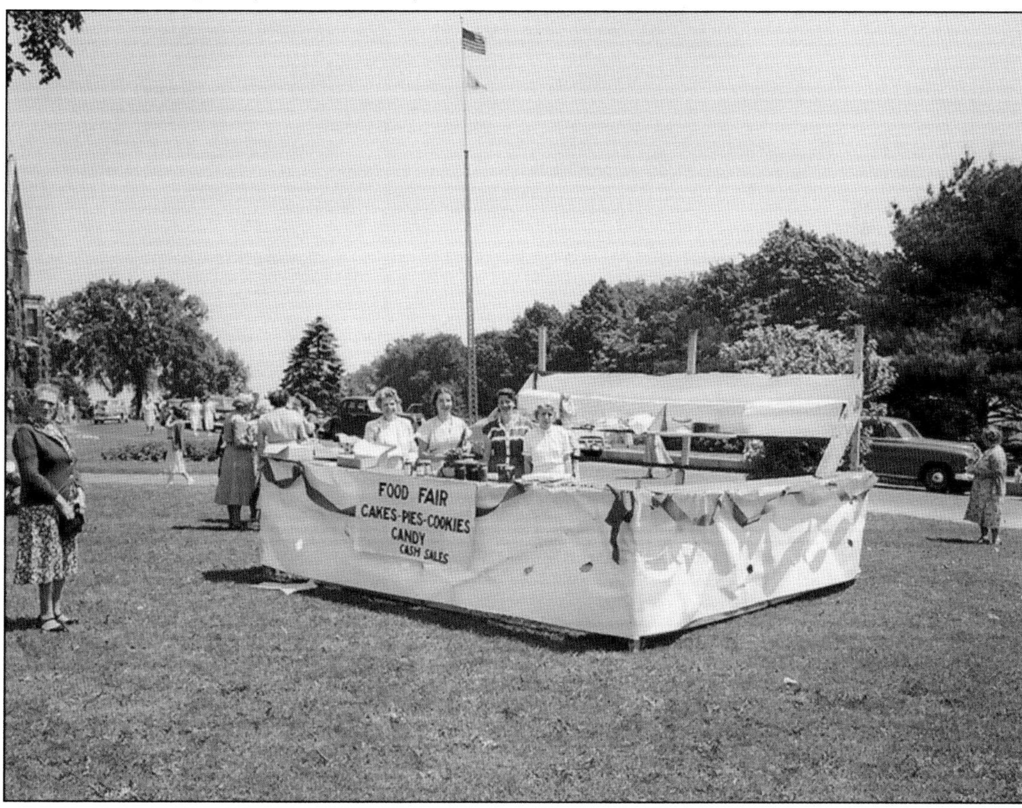
FOOD FAIR
CAKES-PIES-COOKIES
CANDY
CASH SALES

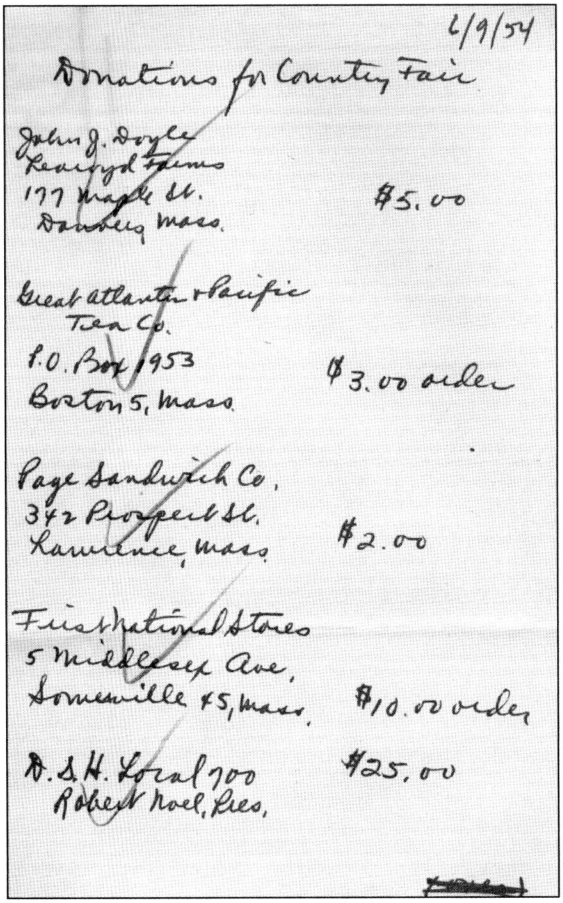

6/9/54

Donations for Country Fair

John J. Doyle
Learoyd Farms
177 Maple St.
Danvers Mass. $5.00

Great Atlantic & Pacific
Tea Co.
P.O. Box 1953
Boston 5, Mass. $3.00 order

Page Sandwich Co.
342 Prospect St.
Lawrence, Mass $2.00

First National Stores
5 Middlesex Ave.
Somerville 45, Mass. $10.00 order

D.S.H. Local 700 $25.00
Robert Noel, Pres.

Large-scale community events like Frontier Day, included local businesses, many of which frequently donated both their time and their wares such as the produce donated by the now defunct Suffolk Farms Packing Co. Included in many of the annual reports issued by the trustees of the asylum were lists of "Gratuitous Services," many of which were donations by locals of magazine subscriptions, money toward patient Christmas gifts, and other small notions that were given by townspeople. Other items, such as snacks for the patients' holiday parties, were supplied by local companies such as the Vincent Potato Chip Company. (Both, David Walsh.)

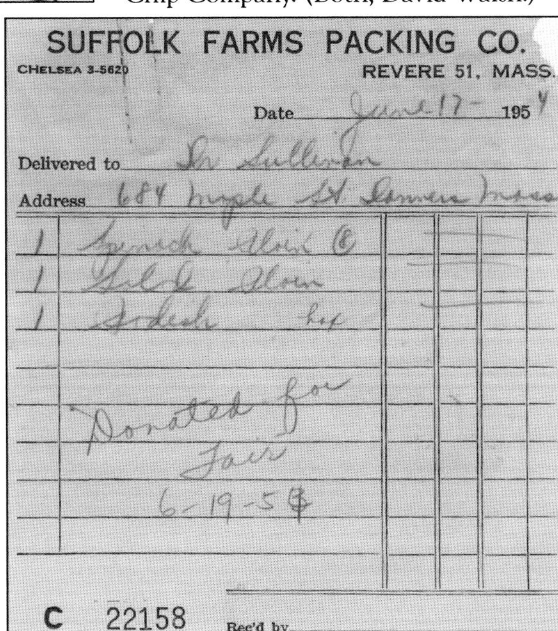

SUFFOLK FARMS PACKING CO.

CHELSEA 3-5620 REVERE 51, MASS.

Date June 17- 1954

Delivered to Dr Sullivan

Address 684 Maple St. Danvers Mass

Donated for Fair 6-19-54

C 22158 Rec'd by

Danvers State Hospital

cordially invites you to attend the

Presentation of Service Awards

and

Reception to the Hospital Volunteers

on Thursday Evening, October 17th, 1957

8:00 to 11:00 p. m.

Hospital Cafeteria

Buffet at conclusion of the program

Danvers State Hospital relied heavily on, and celebrated publicly the service of volunteers who helped plan and run many of the events on the grounds, as well as aid in patient recreational activities. Many came regularly to visit patients and read to them or escort them to activities. They assisted on the wards, helping to run arts and crafts activities or music groups, and they were instrumental in helping special events run smoothly. Those who were not already members of the auxiliary committee would be certain to have the opportunity to enroll at any number of events. (Both, David Walsh.)

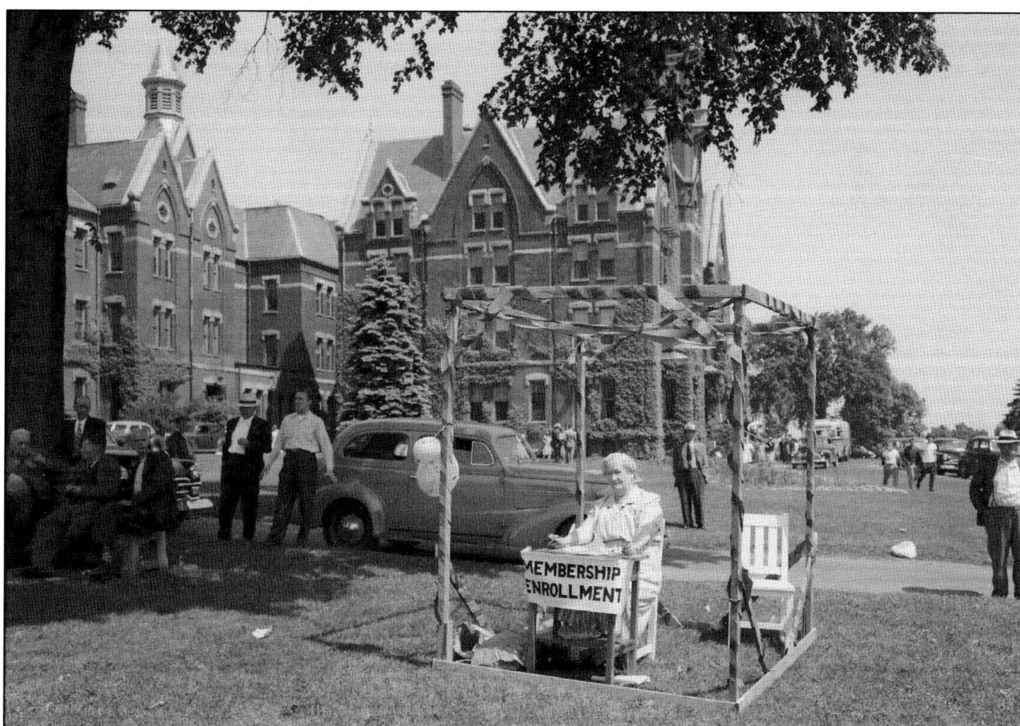

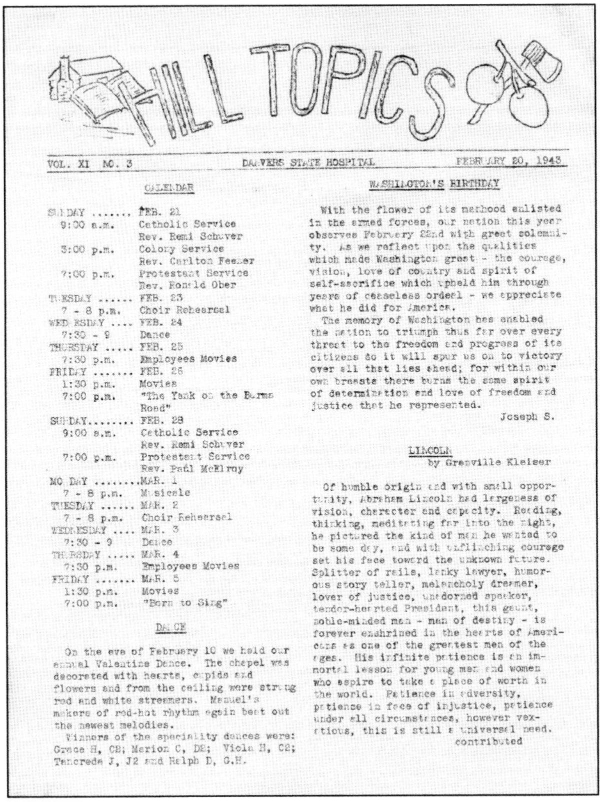

HILL TOPICS

VOL. XI NO. 3 DANVERS STATE HOSPITAL FEBRUARY 20, 1943

CALENDAR

SUNDAY .... FEB. 21
9:00 a.m. Catholic Service
Rev. Remi Schuver
3:00 p.m. Colony Service
Rev. Carlton Feener
7:00 p.m. Protestant Service
Rev. Ronald Ober
TUESDAY ...... FEB. 23
7 - 8 p.m. Choir Rehearsal
WEDNESDAY .... FEB. 24
7:30 - 9 Dance
THURSDAY ..... FEB. 25
7:30 p.m. Employees Movies
FRIDAY .... FEB. 26
1:30 p.m. Movies
7:00 p.m. "The Yank on the Burma Road"
SUNDAY........ FEB. 28
9:00 a.m. Catholic Service
Rev. Remi Schuver
7:00 p.m. Protestant Service
Rev. Paul McElroy
MONDAY ....MAR. 1
7 - 8 p.m. Musicale
TUESDAY ...... MAR. 2
7 - 8 p.m. Choir Rehearsal
WEDNESDAY .... MAR. 3
7:30 - 9 Dance
THURSDAY ..... MAR. 4
7:30 p.m. Employees Movies
FRIDAY .... MAR. 5
1:30 p.m. Movies
7:00 p.m. "Born to Sing"

DANCE

On the eve of February 10 we held our annual Valentine Dance. The chapel was decorated with hearts, cupids and flowers and from the ceiling were strung red and white streamers. Manuel's makers of red-hot rhythm again beat out the newest melodies.

Winners of the speciality dances were: Grace H, C8; Marion C, D8; Viola H, C2; Tancrede J, J2 and Ralph D, G.H.

WASHINGTON'S BIRTHDAY

With the flower of its manhood enlisted in the armed forces, our nation this year observes February 22nd with great solemnity. As we reflect upon the qualities which made Washington great - the courage, vision, love of country and spirit of self-sacrifice which upheld him through years of ceaseless ordeal - we appreciate what he did for America.

The memory of Washington has enabled the nation to triumph thus far over every threat to the freedom and progress of its citizens so it will spur us on to victory over all that lies ahead; for within our own breasts there burns the same spirit of determination and love of freedom and justice that he represented.

Joseph S.

LINCOLN
by Grenville Kleiser

Of humble origin and with small opportunity, Abraham Lincoln had largeness of vision, character and capacity. Reading, thinking, meditating far into the night, he pictured the kind of man he wanted to be some day, and with unflinching courage set his face toward the unknown future. Splitter of rails, lanky lawyer, humorous story teller, melancholy dreamer, lover of justice, unadorned speaker, tender-hearted President, this gaunt, noble-minded man - man of destiny - is forever enshrined in the hearts of Americans as one of the greatest men of the ages. His infinite patience is an immortal lesson for young men and women who aspire to take a place of worth in the world. Patience in adversity, patience in face of injustice, patience under all circumstances, however vexatious, this is still a universal need.

contributed

Throughout its existence, the state hospital produced its own newsletter, *Hill Topics*, which announced events such as religious services, movie showings, and dances. This issue of *Hill Topics*, dated February 20, 1943, even features a patient's writing entitled, "My Cats Teach Me." In later years, the newsletter was renamed *News on the Hill* and was used to communicate important information regarding building closings and patient movements. In the late 1960s, rumors of closure floated around frequently, though very little information was confirmed publicly, lest the hospital lose employees before the official decision had been announced. (Both, David Walsh.)

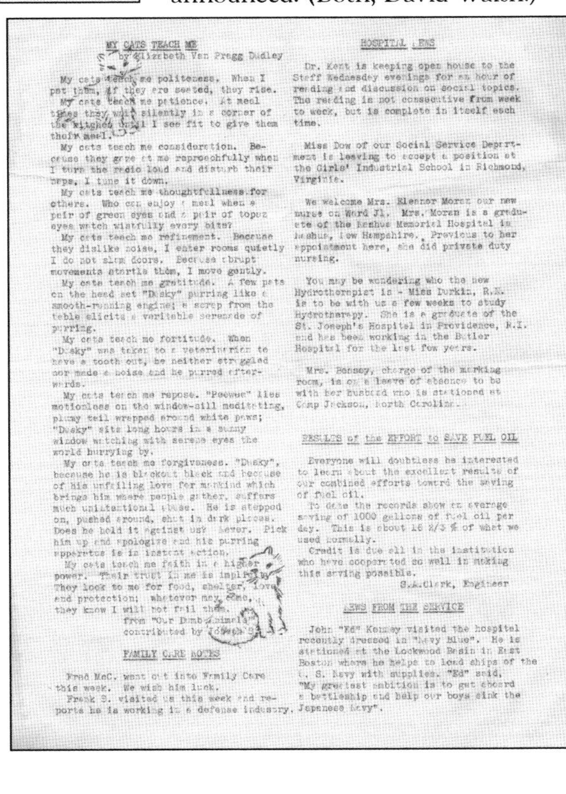

MY CATS TEACH ME
by Elizabeth Van Pragg Dudley

My cats teach me politeness. When I pat them, if they are seated, they rise.

My cats teach me patience. At meal times they wait silently in a corner of the kitchen until I see fit to give them their meal.

My cats teach me consideration. Because they gaze at me reproachfully when I turn the radio loud and disturb their naps, I tune it down.

My cats teach me thoughtfulness for others. Who can enjoy a meal when a pair of green eyes and a pair of topaz eyes watch wistfully every bite?

My cats teach me refinement. Because they dislike noise, I enter rooms quietly I do not slam doors. Because abrupt movements startle them, I move gently.

My cats teach me gratitude. A few pats on the head set "Dusky" purring like a smooth-running engine; a scrap from the table elicits a veritable serenade of purring.

My cats teach me fortitude. When "Dusky" was taken to a veterinarian to have a tooth out, he neither struggled nor made a noise and he purred afterwards.

My cats teach me repose. "Peewee" lies motionless on the window-sill meditating, plumy tail wrapped around white paws; "Dusky" sits long hours in a sunny window watching with serene eyes the world hurrying by.

My cats teach me forgiveness. "Dusky", because he is blackout black and because of his unfailing love for mankind which brings him where people gather, suffers much unintentional abuse. He is stepped on, pushed around, shut in dark places. Does he hold it against us? Never. Pick him up and apologize and his purring apparatus is in instant action.

My cats teach me faith in a higher power. Their trust in me is inspiring. They look to me for food, shelter, love and protection; whatever may come, they know I will not fail them.

from "Our Dumb Animals"
contributed by Joseph S.

FAMILY CARE NOTES

Fred McC. went out into Family Care this week. We wish him luck.

Frank S. visited us this week and reports he is working in a defense industry.

HOSPITAL NEWS

Dr. Kent is keeping open house to the Staff Wednesday evenings for an hour of reading and discussion on social topics. The reading is not consecutive from week to week, but is complete in itself each time.

Miss Dow of our Social Service Department is leaving to accept a position at the Girls' Industrial School in Richmond, Virginia.

We welcome Mrs. Eleanor Moran our new nurse on Ward J1. Mrs. Moran is a graduate of the Nashua Memorial Hospital in Nashua, New Hampshire. Previous to her appointment here, she did private duty nursing.

You may be wondering who the new Hydrotherapist is - Miss Durkin, R.N. is to be with us a few weeks to study Hydrotherapy. She is a graduate of the St. Joseph's Hospital in Providence, R.I. and has been working in the Butler Hospital for the last few years.

Mrs. Bonney, charge of the marking room, is on a leave of absence to be with her husband who is stationed at Camp Jackson, North Carolina.

RESULTS of the EFFORT to SAVE FUEL OIL

Everyone will doubtless be interested to learn about the excellent results of our combined efforts toward the saving of fuel oil.

To date the records show an average saving of 1000 gallons of fuel oil per day. This is about 16 2/3 % of what we used normally.

Credit is due all in the institution who have cooperated so well in making this saving possible.

S.A.Clark, Engineer

NEWS FROM THE SERVICE

John "Ed" Kenney visited the hospital recently dressed in "Navy Blue". He is stationed at the Lockwood Basin in East Boston where he helps to load ships of the U. S. Navy with supplies. "Ed" said, "My greatest ambition is to get aboard a battleship and help our boys sink the Japanese Navy".

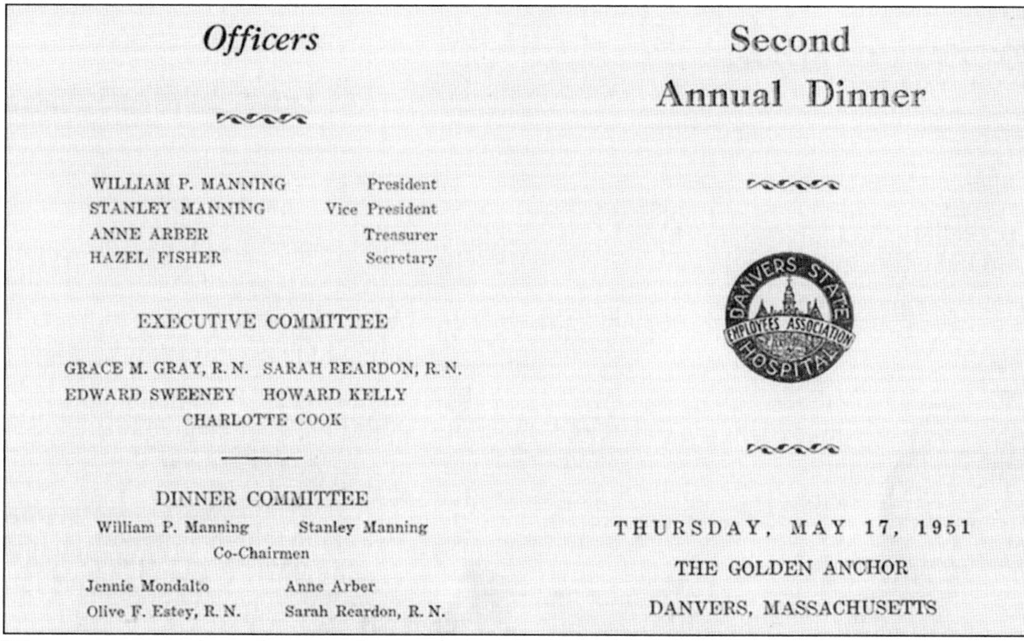

Officers

WILLIAM P. MANNING — President
STANLEY MANNING — Vice President
ANNE ARBER — Treasurer
HAZEL FISHER — Secretary

EXECUTIVE COMMITTEE

GRACE M. GRAY, R. N. SARAH REARDON, R. N.
EDWARD SWEENEY HOWARD KELLY
CHARLOTTE COOK

DINNER COMMITTEE

William P. Manning Stanley Manning
Co-Chairmen

Jennie Mondalto Anne Arber
Olive F. Estey, R. N. Sarah Reardon, R. N.

Second
Annual Dinner

THURSDAY, MAY 17, 1951
THE GOLDEN ANCHOR
DANVERS, MASSACHUSETTS

This is a program from the second annual Danvers State Hospital Employees Association Dinner held May 17, 1951, at the now defunct Golden Anchor in Danvers. At the height of its census, hospital staff cared for over 2,500 patients at any given time in a building originally built to house only 450. (John Gray.)

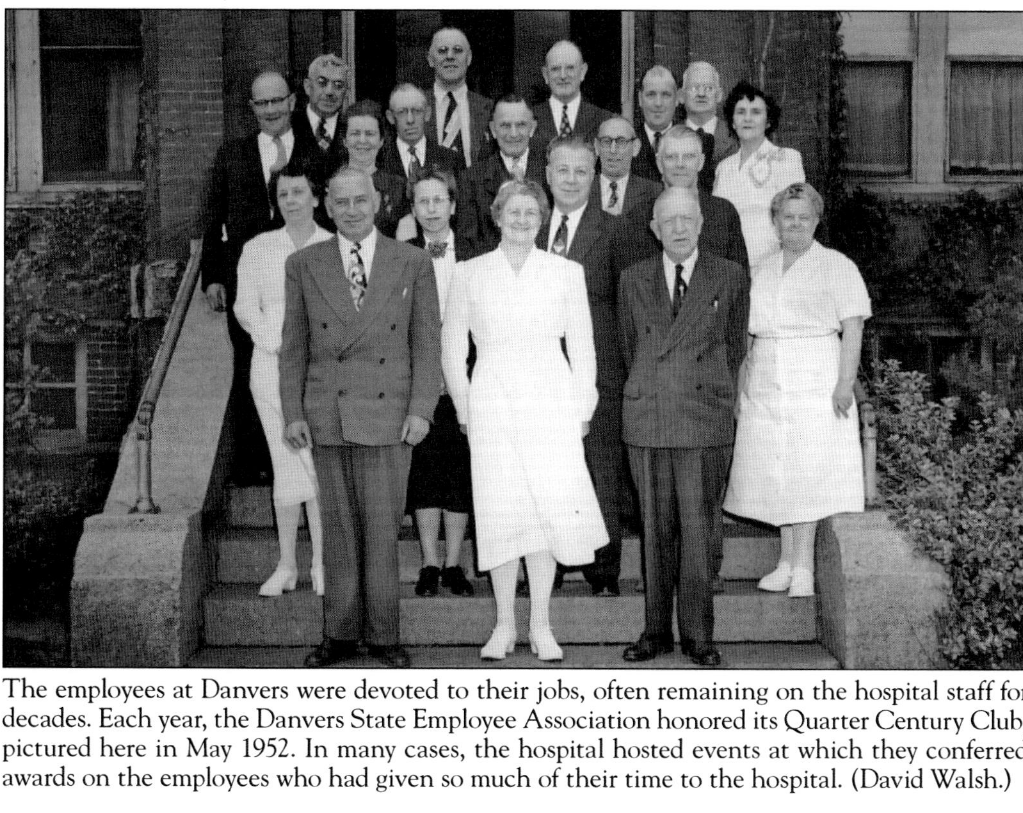

The employees at Danvers were devoted to their jobs, often remaining on the hospital staff for decades. Each year, the Danvers State Employee Association honored its Quarter Century Club, pictured here in May 1952. In many cases, the hospital hosted events at which they conferred awards on the employees who had given so much of their time to the hospital. (David Walsh.)

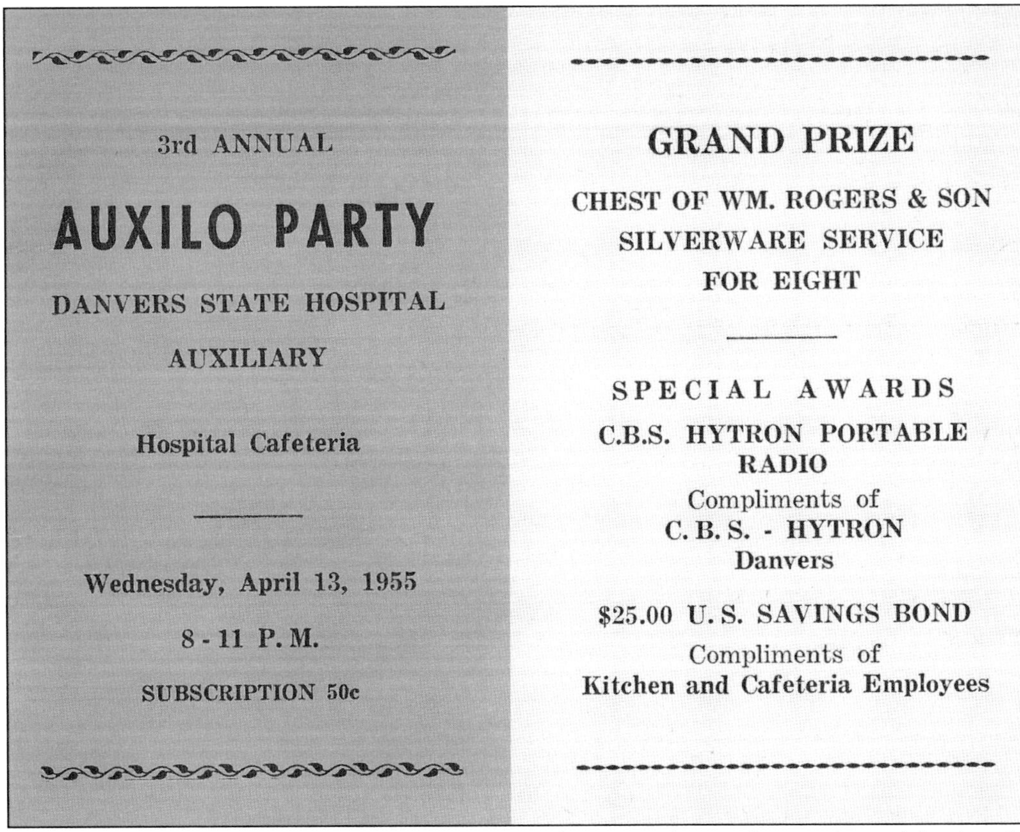

3rd ANNUAL

AUXILO PARTY

DANVERS STATE HOSPITAL

AUXILIARY

Hospital Cafeteria

Wednesday, April 13, 1955

8 - 11 P. M.

SUBSCRIPTION 50c

GRAND PRIZE

CHEST OF WM. ROGERS & SON
SILVERWARE SERVICE
FOR EIGHT

SPECIAL AWARDS

C.B.S. HYTRON PORTABLE
RADIO
Compliments of
C. B. S. - HYTRON
Danvers

$25.00 U. S. SAVINGS BOND
Compliments of
Kitchen and Cafeteria Employees

The Danvers State Hospital Auxiliary hosted annual events to honor the members of the Auxilo. This program from the third annual Auxilo party on April 13, 1955, was held in the hospital cafeteria and boasted prizes such as silverware service for eight, a portable radio, and a $25 US savings bond, all of which were raffled off at the event. (Amanda Kohut.)

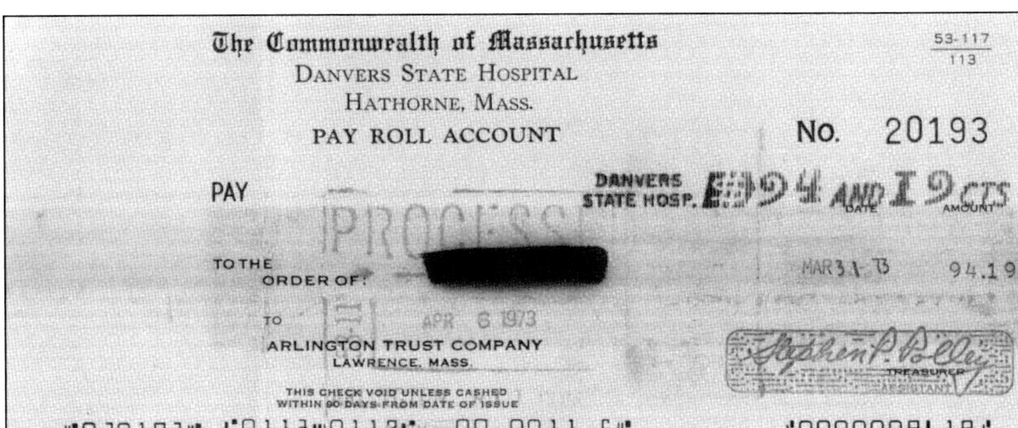

The Commonwealth of Massachusetts
DANVERS STATE HOSPITAL
HATHORNE, MASS.
PAY ROLL ACCOUNT

53-117
113

No. 20193

PAY DANVERS STATE HOSP. $94 AND 19 CTS

TO THE ORDER OF

MAR 31 73 94.19

TO ARLINGTON TRUST COMPANY
LAWRENCE, MASS.

THIS CHECK VOID UNLESS CASHED WITHIN 90 DAYS FROM DATE OF ISSUE

TREASURER

By 1973, the average weekly wage was $157. As budget cuts continued and funding was reduced, staff at Danvers State Hospital felt the pinch as well; for example, this paycheck shows an employee earning less than the median salary rate. Boxes of canceled paychecks were left behind in the offices of the Kirkbride when it closed. (Jett Chapman.)

Four

DECLINE AND LOSS

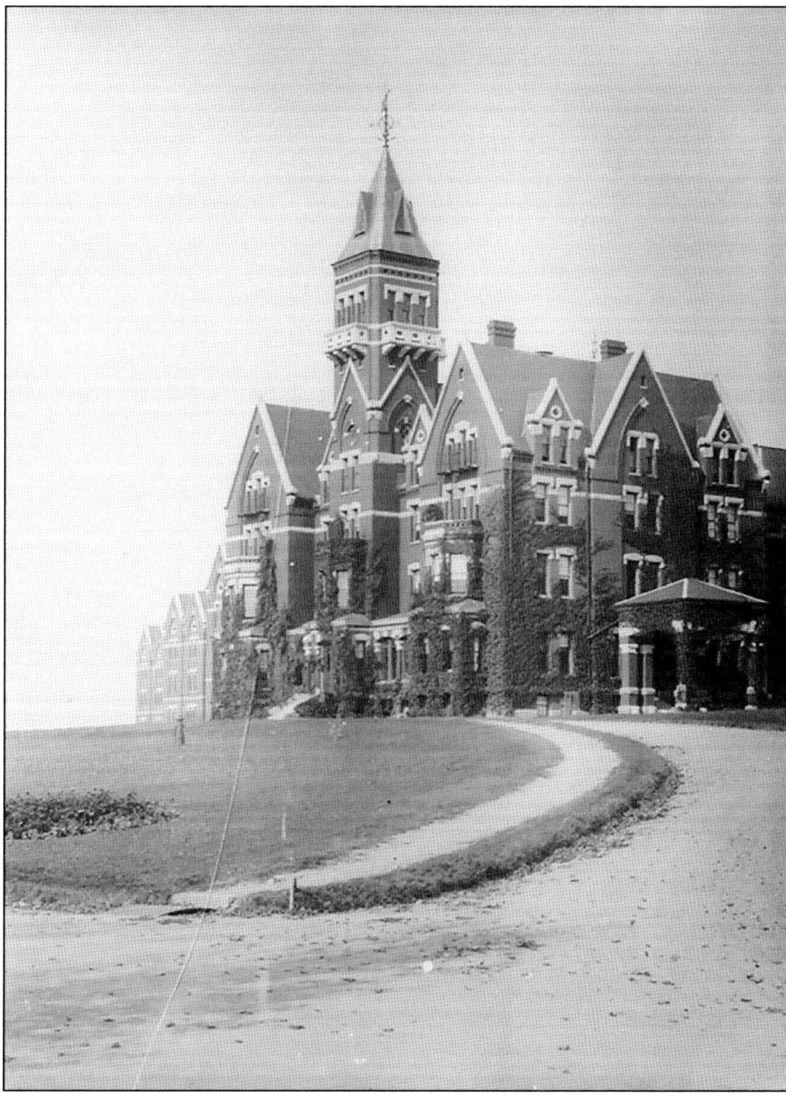

Escapes were recorded at the state hospital as early as 1880, when Charles Freeman, the "child butcherer" disappeared from the institution. Another made headlines in 1920 when a young woman, charged with fraud, escaped from Danvers. Later, escapes would be recorded once a month on average, though most were repeats. (John Gray.)

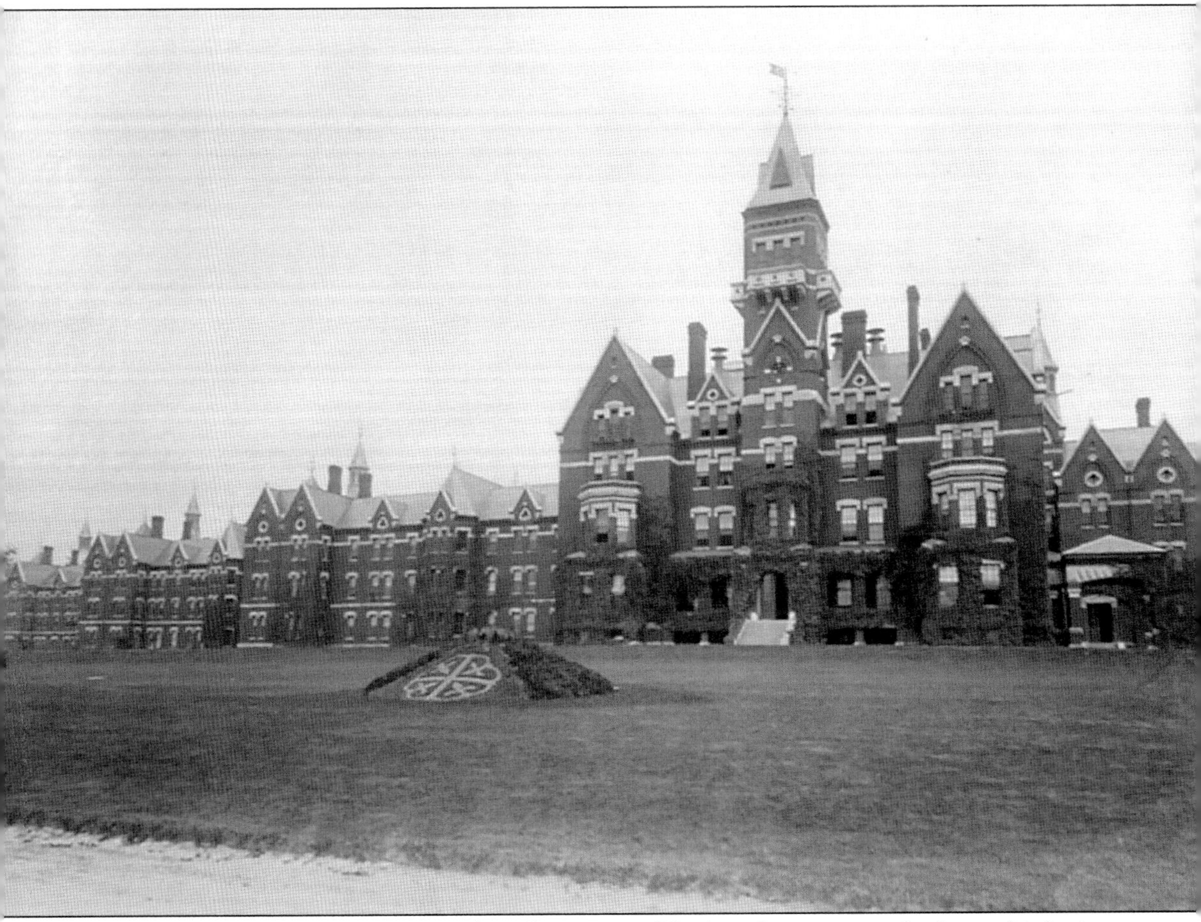

A number of fires were also reported on the campus. The laundry room caught fire multiple times in spite of new equipment, as recorded in the annual report of 1901. Two major fires destroyed a great deal of hospital property in 1912. On January 24, a fire destroyed a ventilation tower and a considerable portion of the roof. One person was injured after falling from a staircase. A second fire on October 25 destroyed a barn at Middleton Colony. (John Gray.)

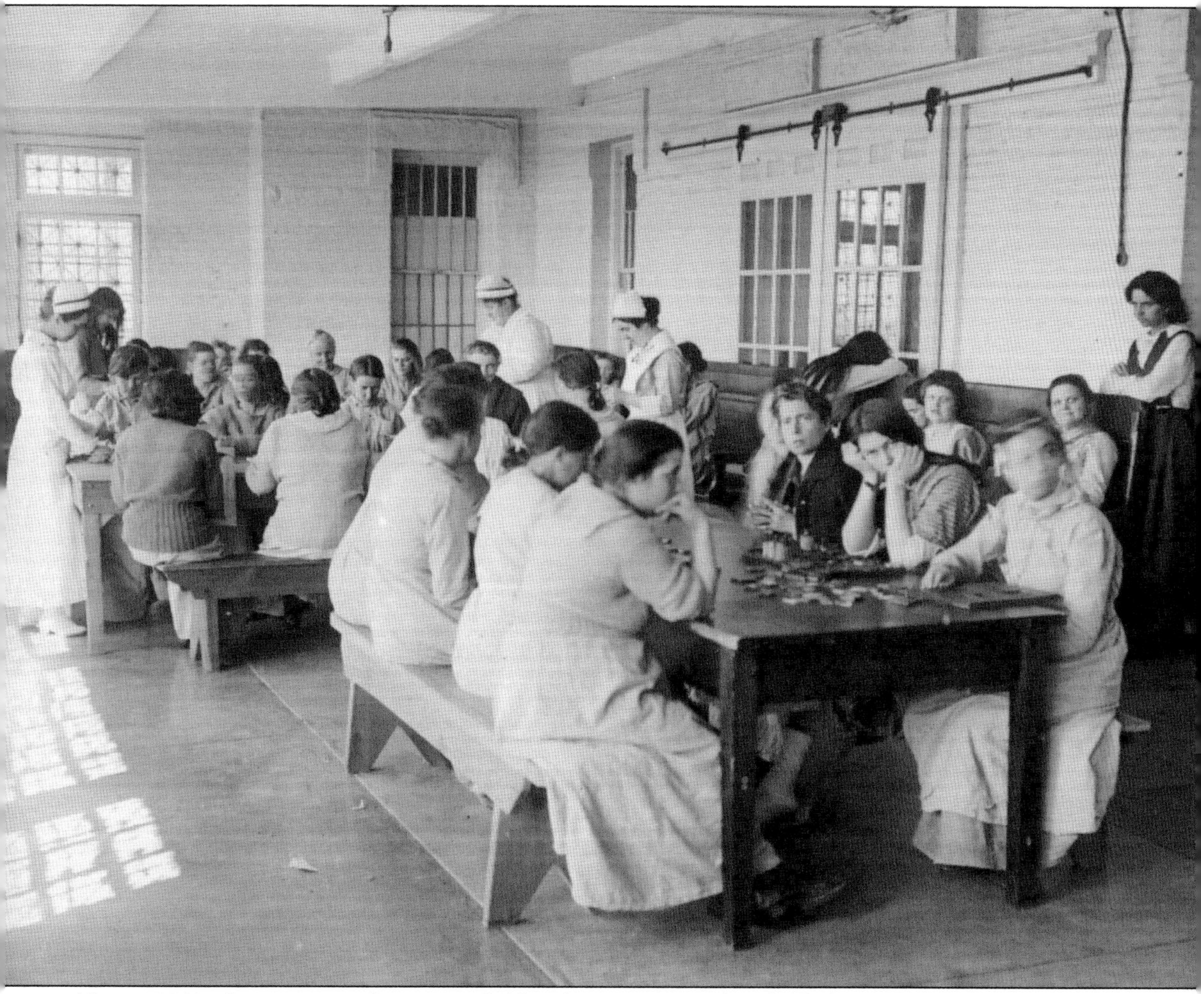

Also in 1912, the position of eugenics fieldworker was created and filled in an effort to reach out to and study the families of those committed to Danvers State Hospital. Eugenicists believed that the traits causing insanity and low moral behavior were a matter of heredity and could be studied in previous generations. (Ben Kenny.)

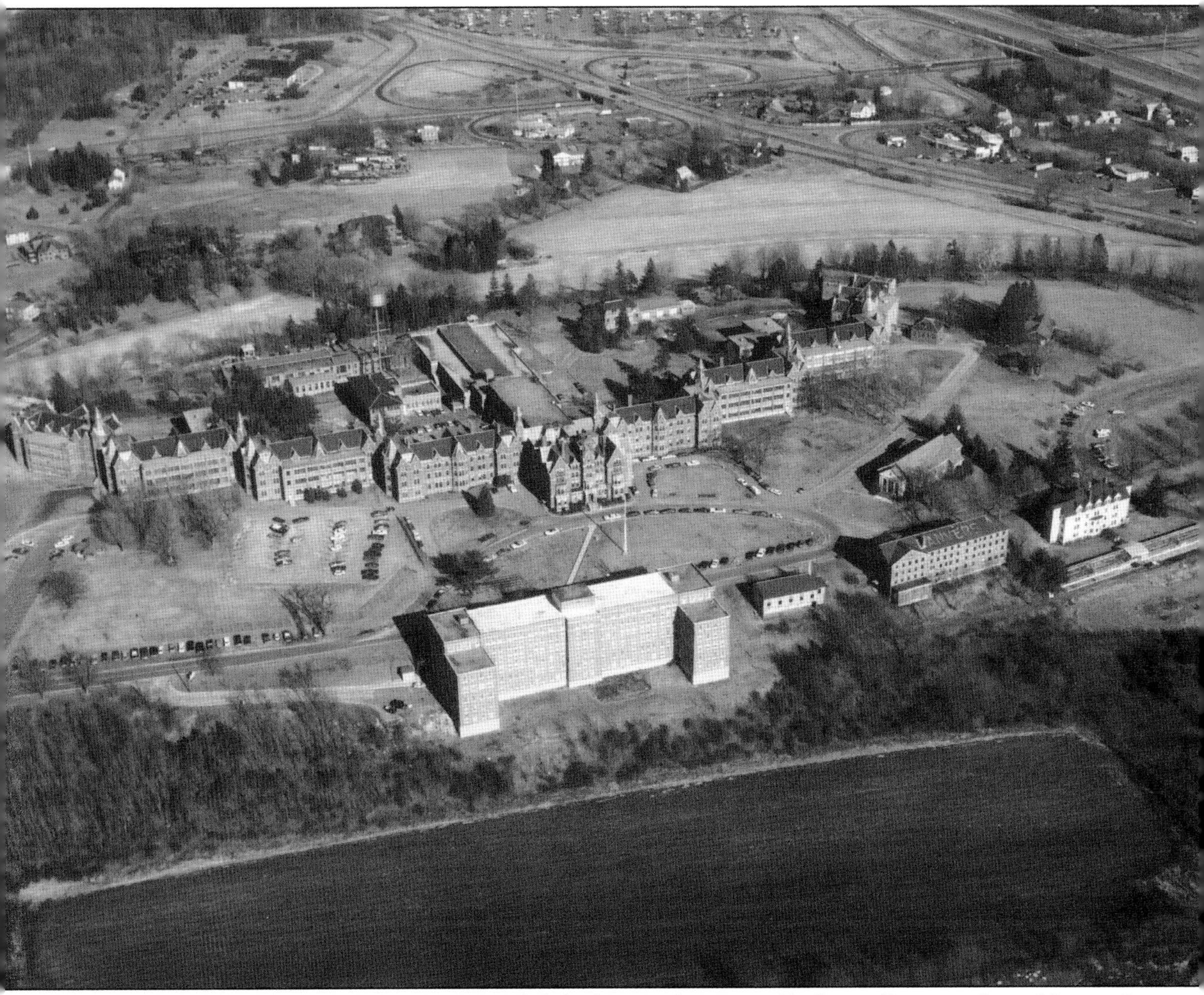

As the patient population grew, so too did the hospital campus. Early on, Danvers State Hospital had moved away from the Kirkbride model and expanded into what was referred to as the "colony" model, with numerous buildings on campus serving multiple purposes; first with the addition of the Bonner Building and later with construction of the Hogan Building, known as the Hathorne State School. The campus then spread farther, down to the lowlands where patients lived in farm buildings so they could be closer to their work. This movement would eventually make it easier for the state to empty out the main Kirkbride, relocating patients and offices to the Bonner Building. Eventually, it too would close, with patients moving out to the community instead. Only Hogan would remain in operation. (Massachusetts Archives.)

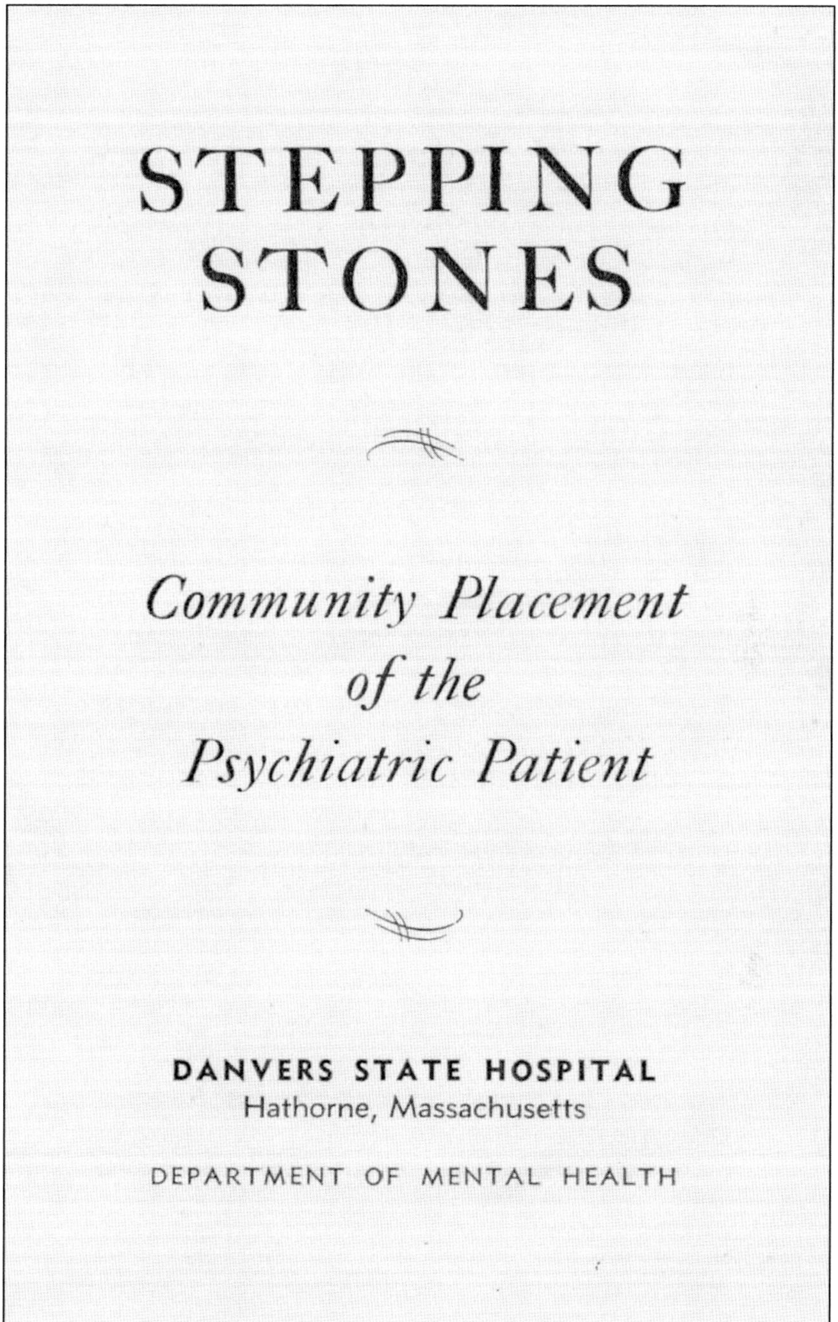

STEPPING STONES

Community Placement of the Psychiatric Patient

DANVERS STATE HOSPITAL
Hathorne, Massachusetts

DEPARTMENT OF MENTAL HEALTH

Beginning in the early 1970s, there was a shift in treatment focus from institutionalization to community treatment in group homes and outpatient programs. The patient population at Danvers plummeted from a high of 2,600 to only 260 as the hospital was phased out. Hospital operations were moved from the main Kirkbride to the Bonner Building, and the Kirkbride was left abandoned. The entire campus was declared to be "surplus property" by the state in 1998, and the then Department of Capital Asset Management put out a request for development proposals. (Amanda Kohut.)

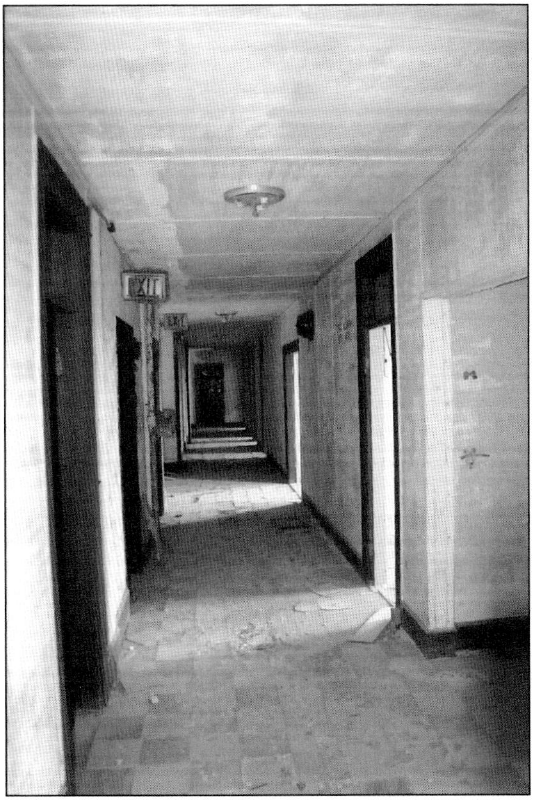

The first efforts to establish community treatment of the mentally ill were made in the 1920s and 1930s, though asylum populations continued to grow. With the advent of antipsychotics such as chlorpromazine, also known as Thorazine, a greater push toward deinstitutionalization was made beginning in the 1960s. By the 1980s, multiple lawsuits were brought against institutions nationwide, resulting in changes to the commitment process as well as treatment models. At one time, the seven state hospitals operating in Massachusetts served upwards of 25,000 patients. By the late 1980s, that number had dropped to 2,500, with the majority of the patients transferred into community mental health treatment. (Both, John Archer.)

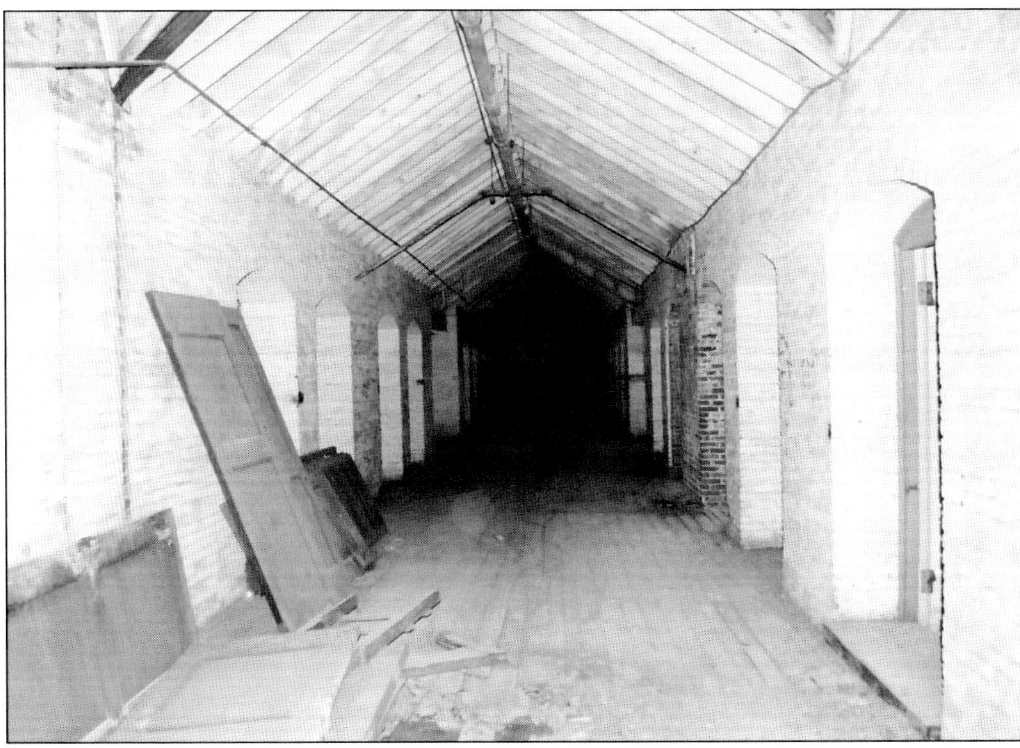

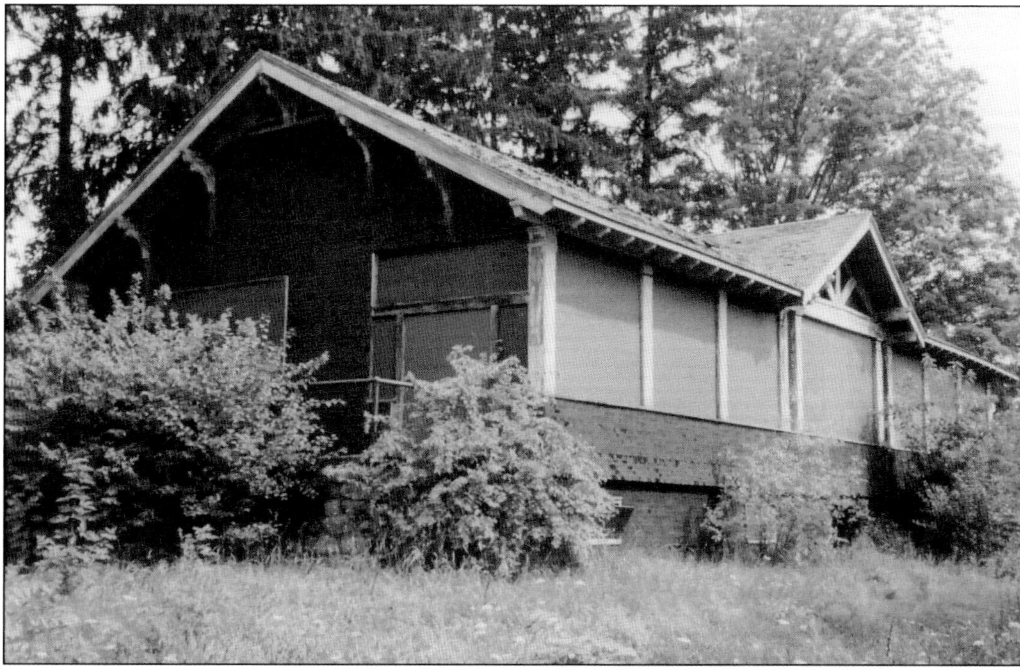

In 1908, French scientists Albert Calmette and Camille Guerin set out to develop a vaccine for tuberculosis, developing the BCG vaccine, which was officially introduced in 1921. By 1944, antibiotics were also developed for use against tuberculosis. Eventually, it was believed that the disease had been eradicated and hospital administrators decided that they no longer needed separate containment and treatment facilities. The small TB cottages at the outskirts of the campus were converted into art and music cottages for group therapy. Both are pictured here abandoned, long after they fell out of use. (Above, John Archer; below, John Gray.)

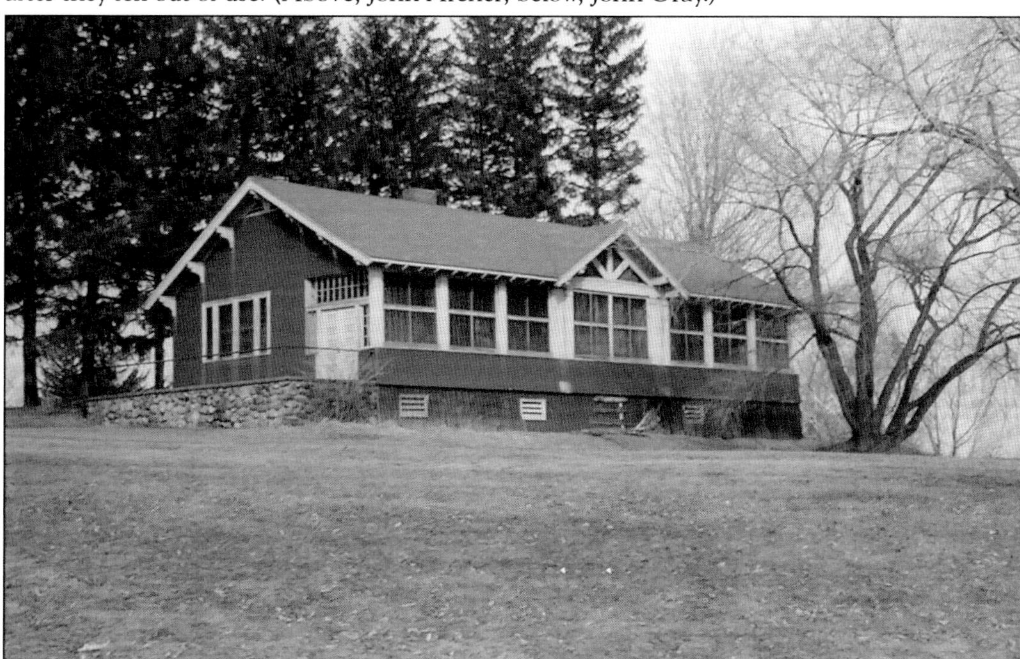

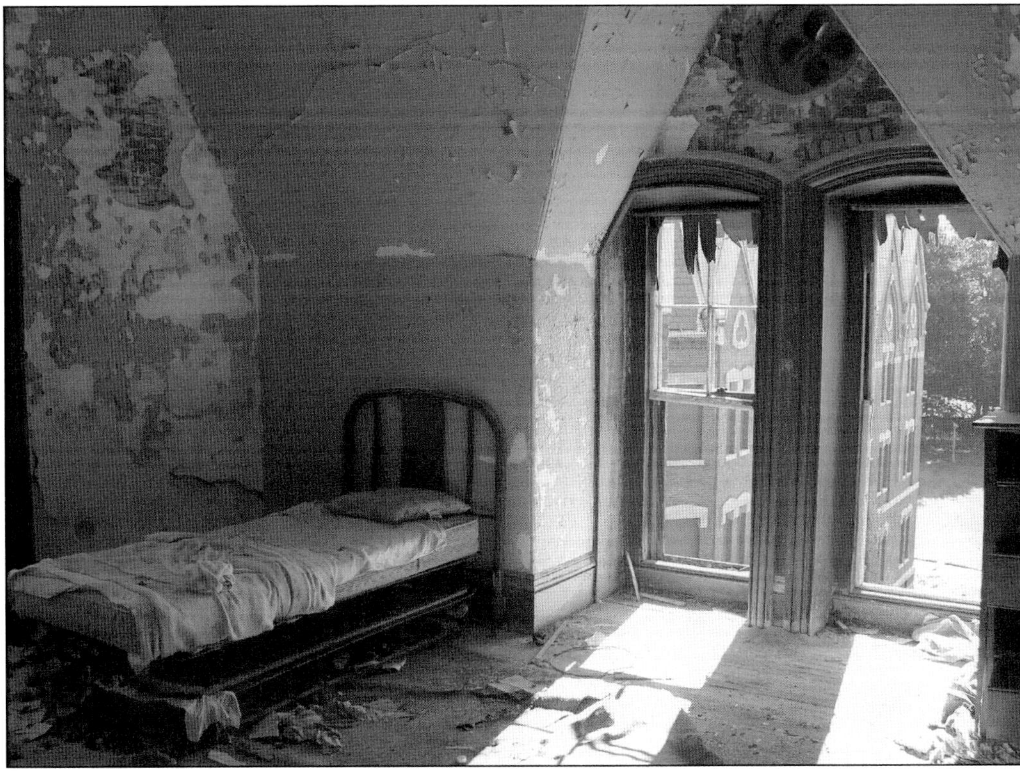

Danvers State Hospital closed its doors for good after the last patients and staff were transferred to Tewksbury State Hospital on June 24, 1992. Members of the maintenance staff went from building to building locking the doors along with the assistant superintendent, hospital administrators, and campus police. The hospital would sit, abandoned and decaying, for more than 10 years. Due in large part to its reputation and the lore surrounding the hospital, the property attracted scores of urban explorers and photographers, like John Gray, who had the opportunity to photograph the building as it decayed. Pictured here are images Gray recorded of the asylum and its wards, which are included in his book *Abandoned Asylums of New England*. (John Gray.)

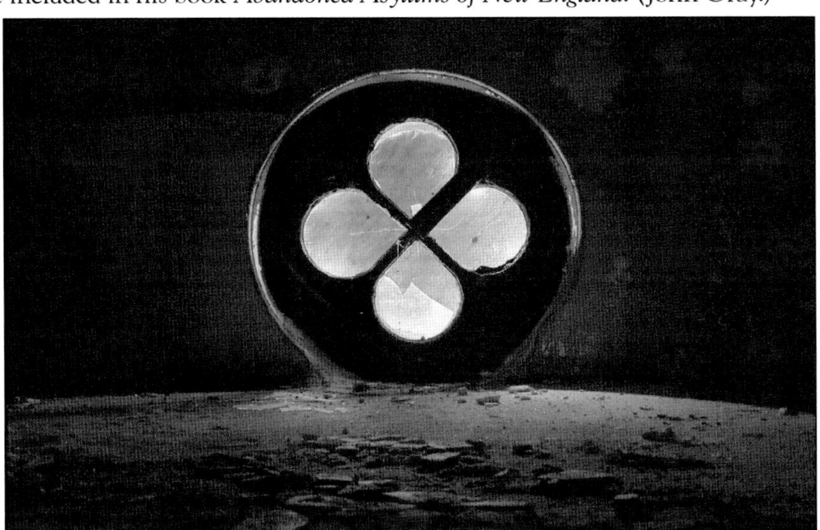

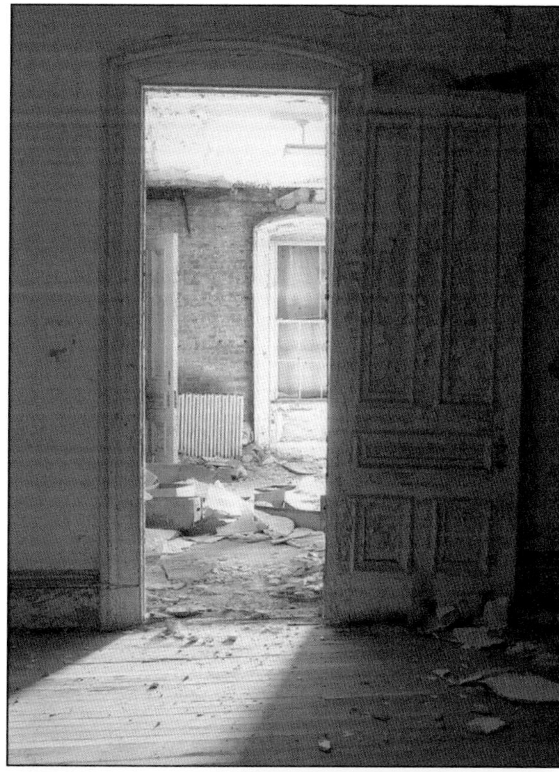

Urban exploration, the exploration of abandoned man-made structures, led to thorough documentation of many of the abandoned asylums across the United States, but most especially Danvers State Hospital. In the years that it was abandoned, many renowned photographers chronicled the building in varying states of decay. Websites sprang up featuring images of Danvers, some with copious amounts of historical information about the asylum. John Gray's website, Danvers State Insane Asylum (www.danversstateinsaneasylum.com), became one of the most comprehensive resources on Danvers. It features a rare glimpse into the closed world of the state hospital. (Both, John Gray.)

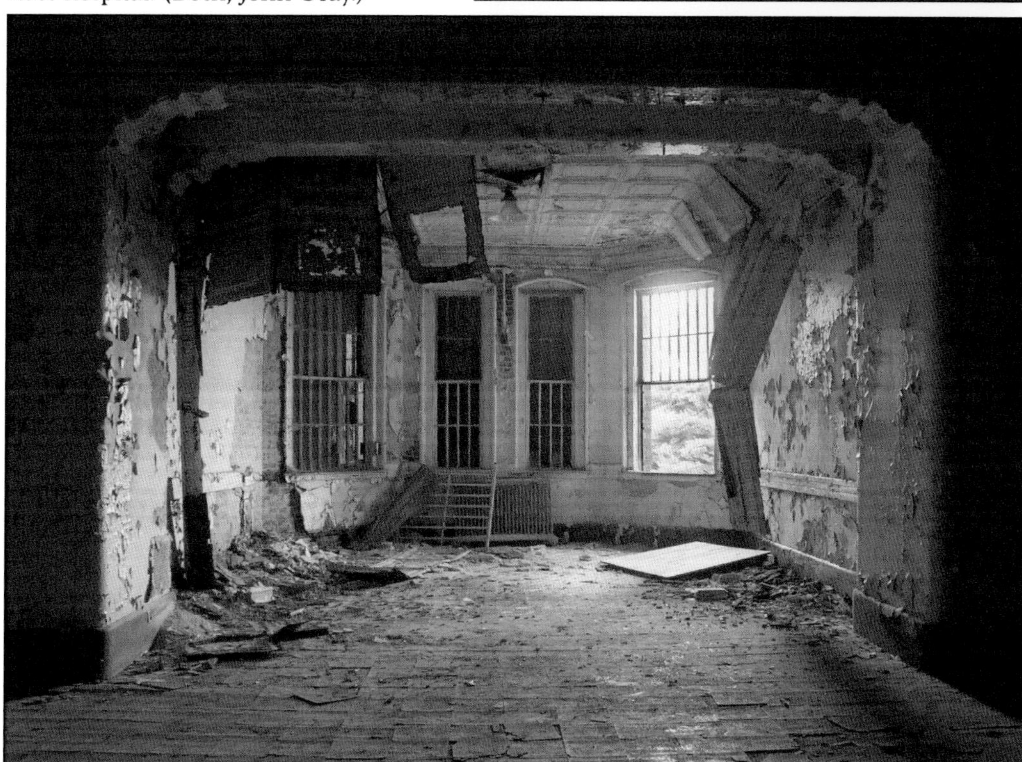

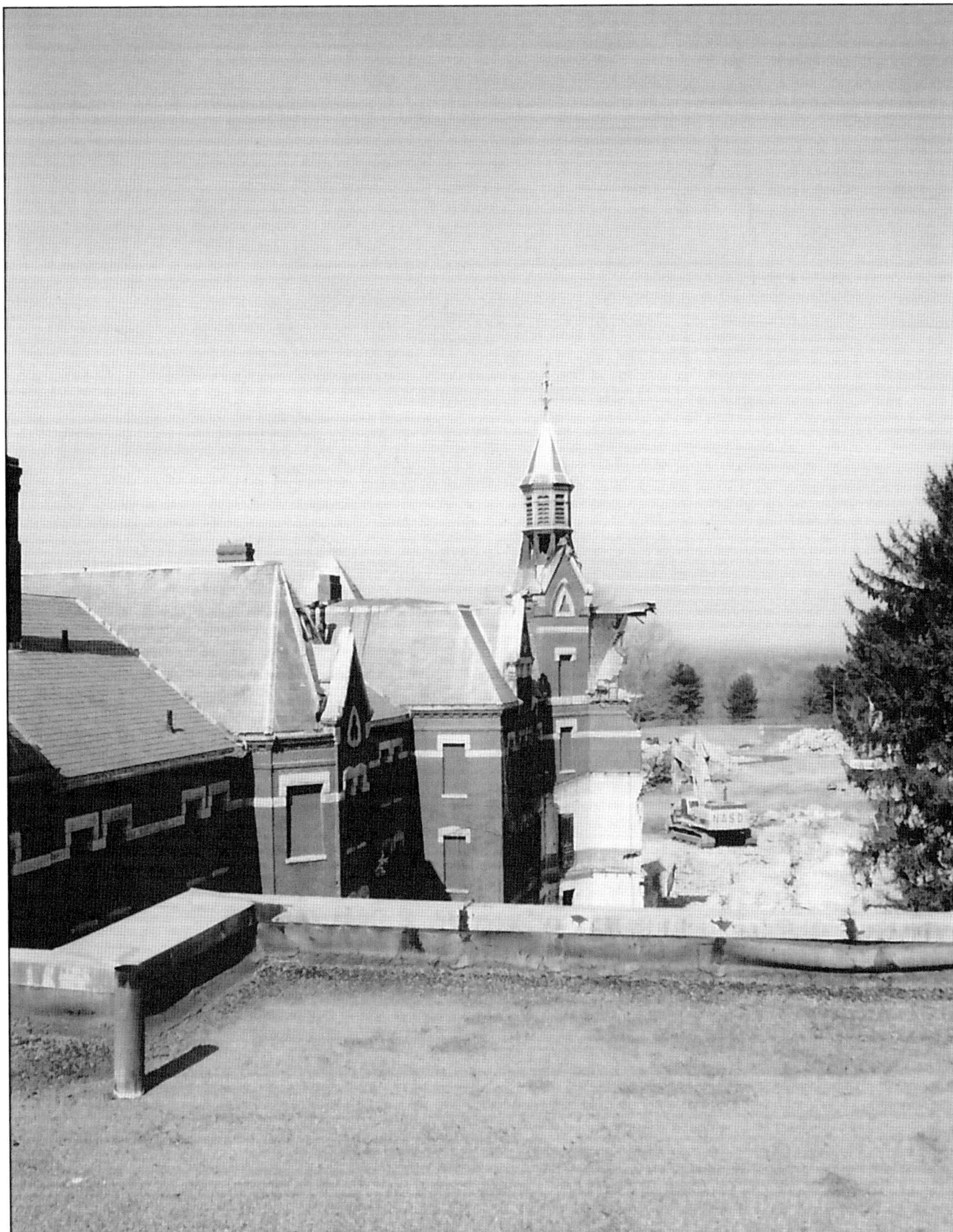

In the annual report issued in 1989, it was clear that the staff of Danvers State Hospital held out hope that it would remain in operation. Under the supervision of a medical director rather than a superintendent, two additional psychiatrists were hired and six more rotated in from other hospitals. They planned to continue recruiting staff well into 1990. Though they were continuing to provide patients with community treatment opportunities, the hospital administration remained focused on the future and set lofty goals for the next fiscal year. In spite of all the positive changes that had been made at Danvers, the state decided in 1991 to close the hospital for good. (John Archer.)

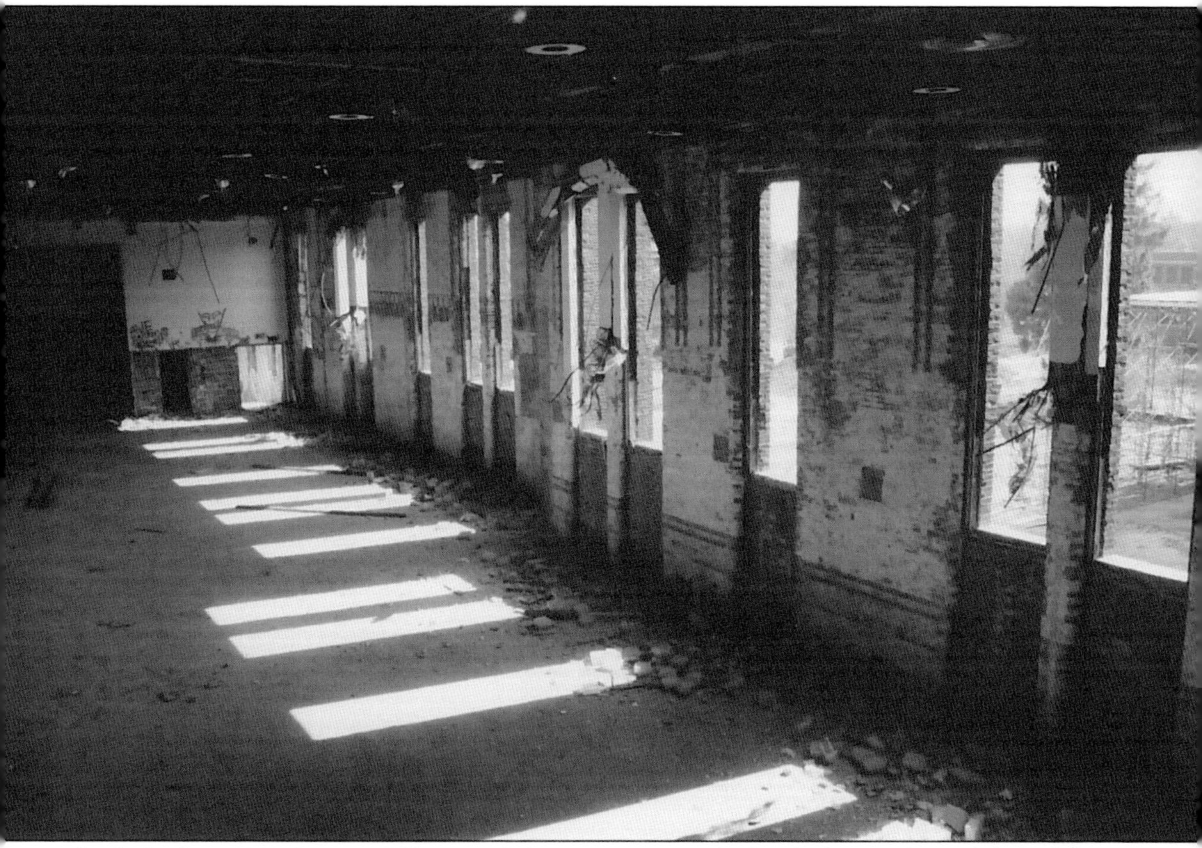

As far back as 1982, Lozano, White, and Associates were asked to look into the viability of the Kirkbride. Their report deemed the entire hospital complex to be of major historical significance and suggested it be retained in its entirety. The same firm would later present a similar report for Northampton State Hospital. After having written her thesis on the state hospital in 1981, architecture student Marcia Cini petitioned for the hospital campus to be added to the National Historic Register. Her thesis, *The Hospital Palace*, was instrumental in recording the history of the state hospital. (John Archer.)

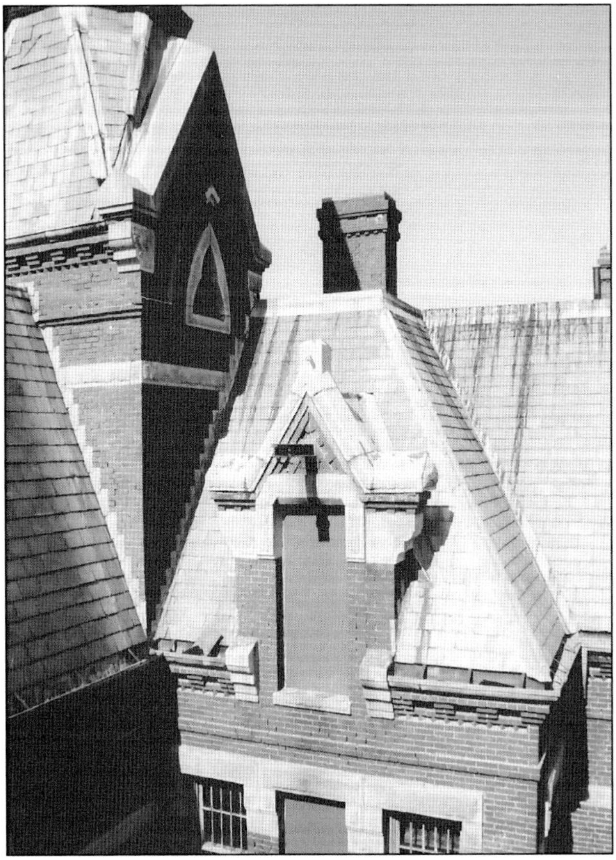

The first developer to enter into negotiations with the State of Massachusetts was Archstone Communities. The company released its plans for redevelopment to the historic commission and other interested parties in early 2002. After numerous discussions about the historical significance of the Danvers State Hospital campus, Archstone Communities presented a development plan that directly contradicted its early promises to retain the majority of the Kirkbride and instead called for the demolition of four wards. At the last minute, Archstone Communities withdrew its redevelopment plans and the project ground to a halt. Another year would go by before any changes would be made on Hathorne Hill. (Both, John Archer.)

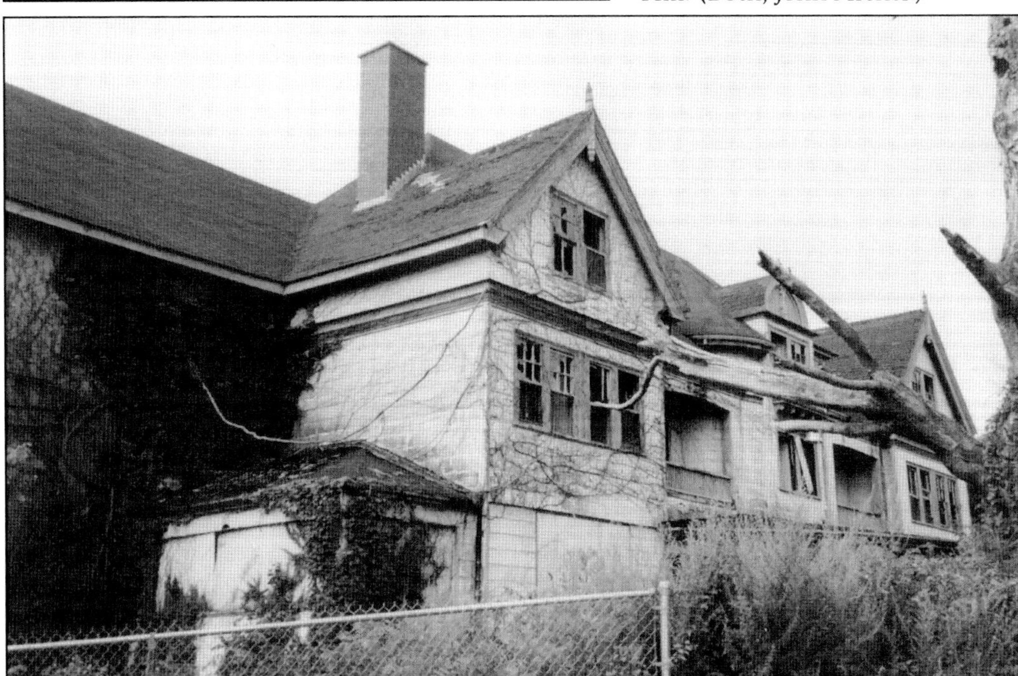

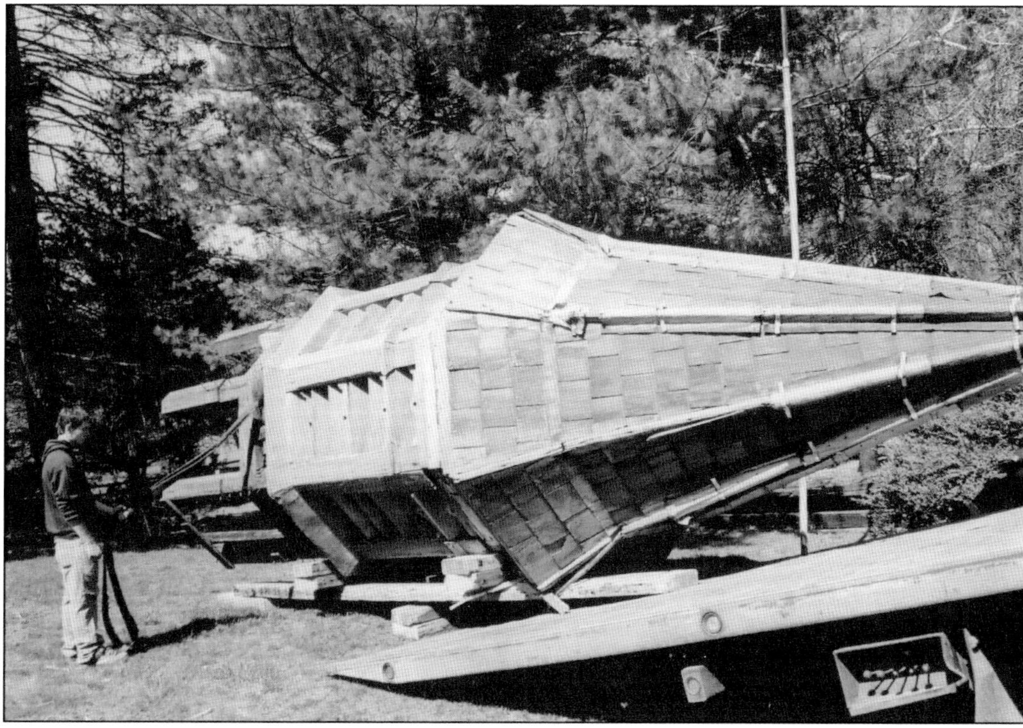

In 2003 Boston area developer AvalonBay picked up where Archstone left off and submitted an application for demolition of certain parts of the state hospital as part of its redevelopment plan. The application would allow AvalonBay to demolish Wards A, B, I, and J on either side of the administration building. Pictured above is an image of the spire from Ward H after it was removed, waiting to be taken to the home of Danvers resident John Archer, who would later build an addition to his home, of which the spire is its centerpiece. (Above, John Archer; below, photograph by Katherine Anderson.)

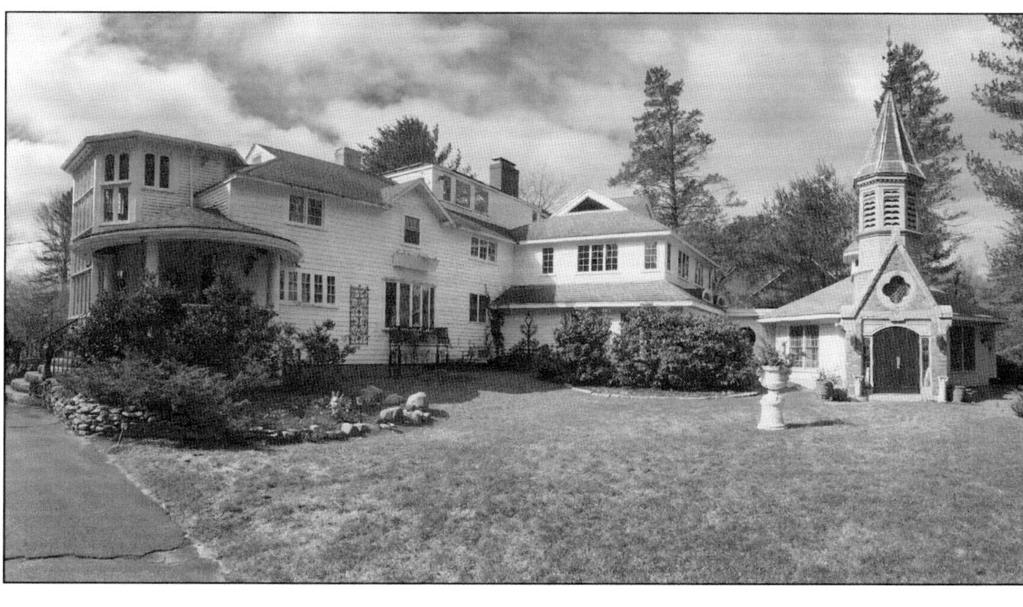

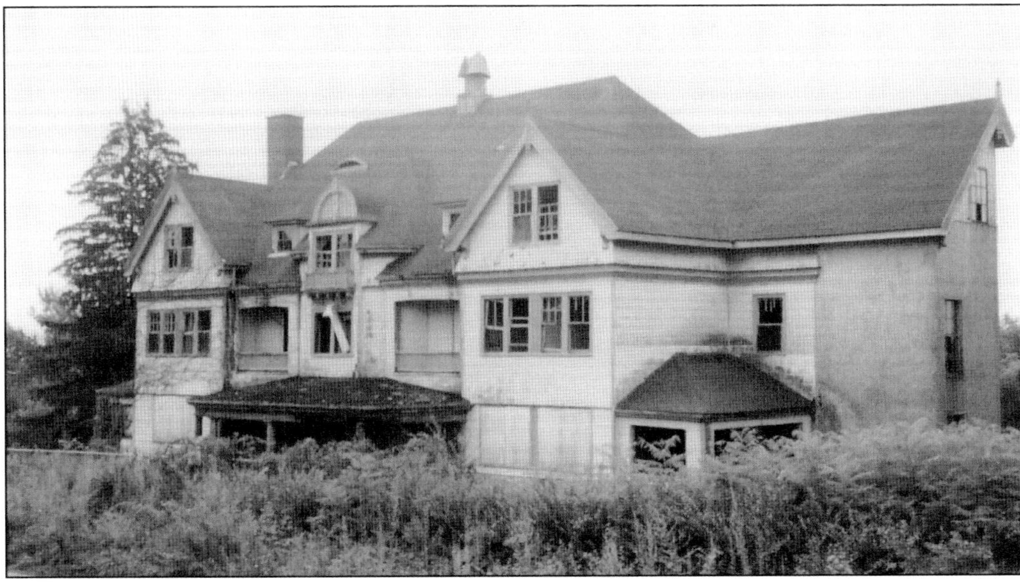

John Archer, a local businessman and member of the Danvers Historical Society, attended a campus walkthrough with the developers and archivist Richard Trask of the Peabody Library. Together, they helped to catalog the remaining buildings, most of which had been added to the National Historic Register yet were still slated for demolition. The images taken on that walkthrough were assembled into a portfolio of sorts that is now all that remains of the campus in its entirety. Pictured here is Gray Gables along with an example of the covered staircases that dotted the rear of the Kirkbride. (Above, John Archer; below, Danvers Archival Center, Danvers, Massachusetts.)

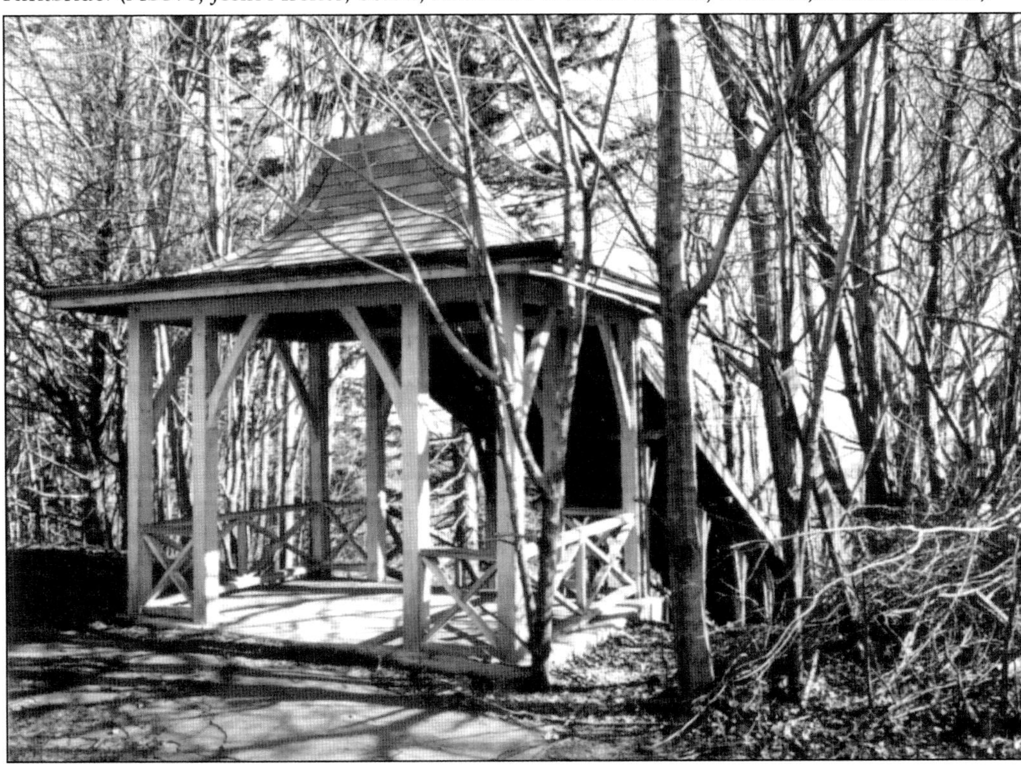

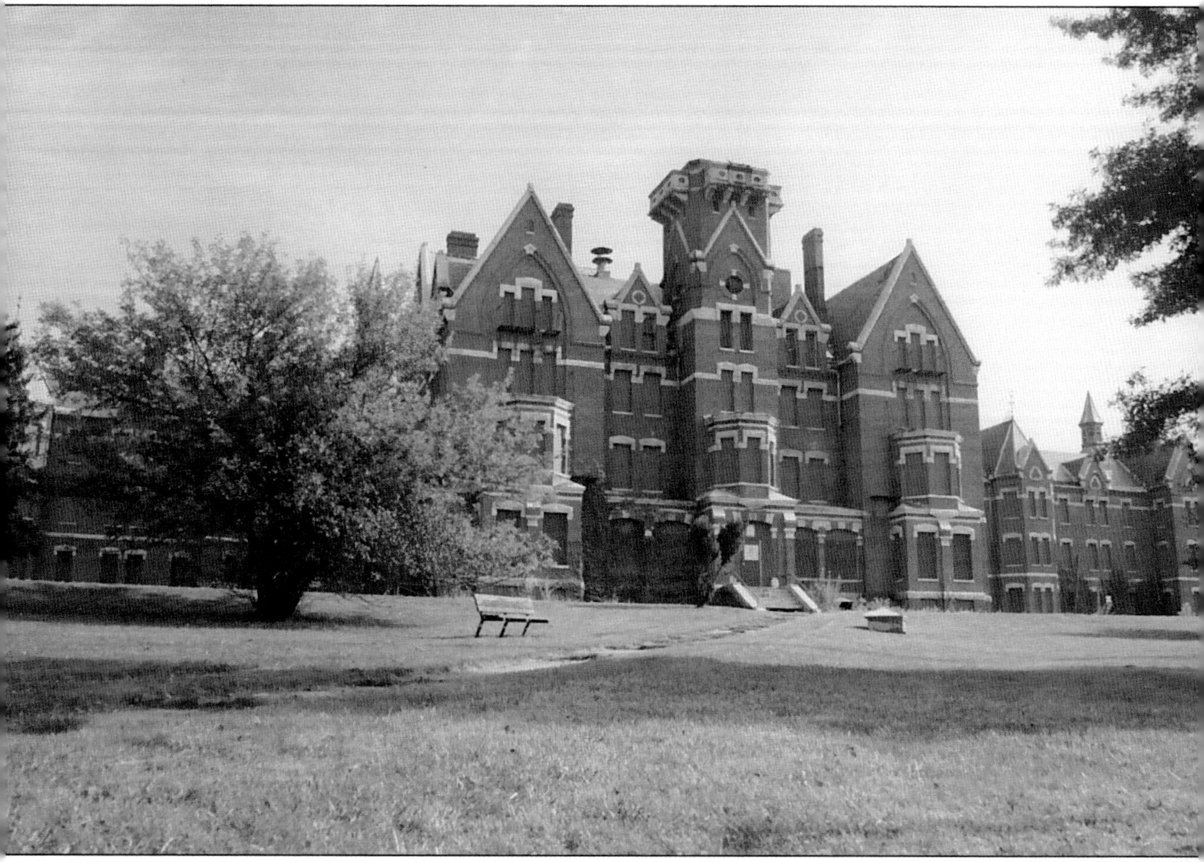

This photograph of Danvers State Hospital, taken a number of years before demolition, is one of the most iconic photographs taken while it was still abandoned. This view features heavily in the film *Session 9* and is likely one of the most recognizable images of the Kirkbride. In spite of the boards on the lower windows, there were many open spaces that left the building vulnerable to the elements, including the harsh New England winters. The boards also did little to keep explorers, vandals, and scrappers from going through the building; in some cases, doing far more damage to the building than the weather ever could, including a few reported cases of arson. (John Archer.)

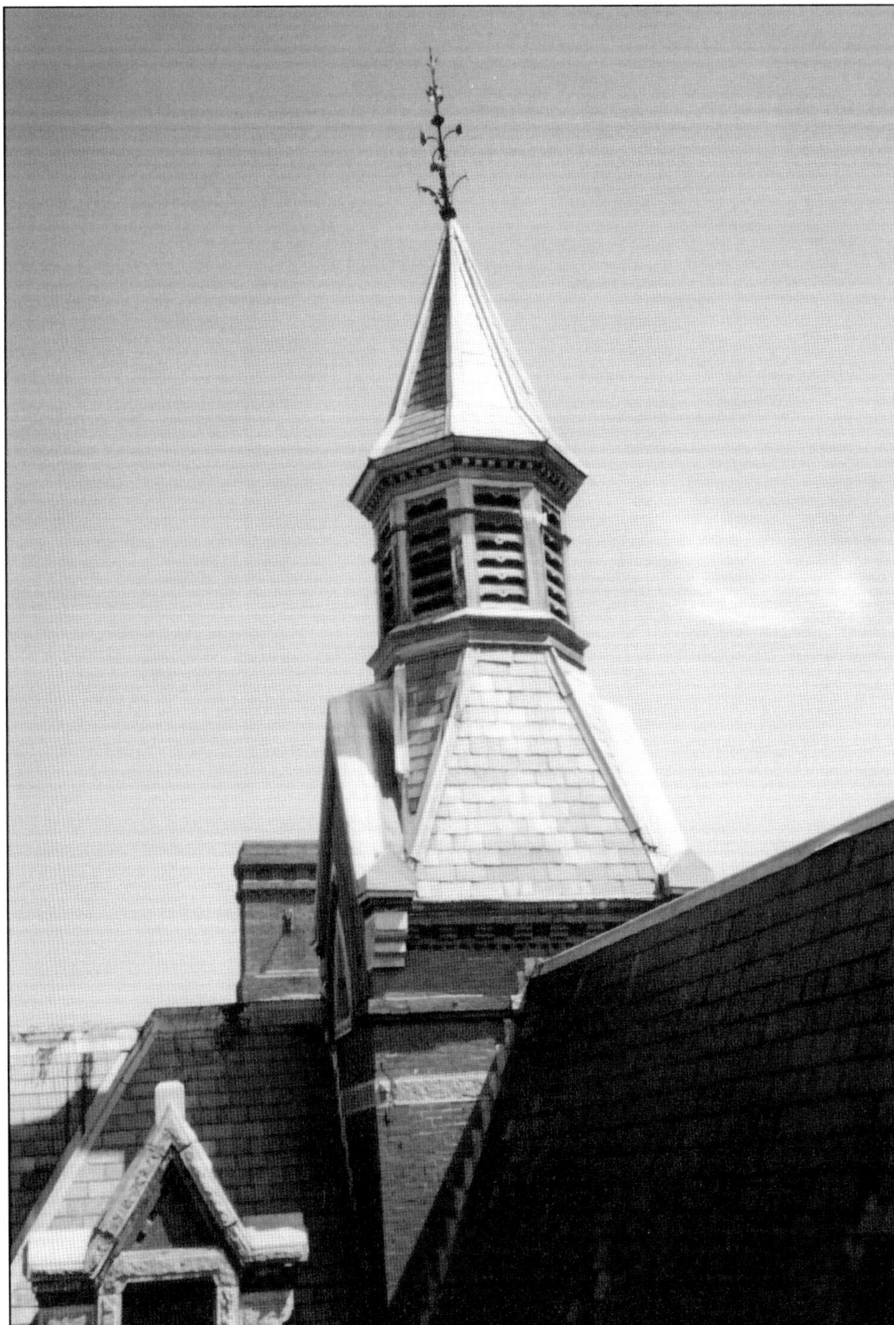

As demolition began, a number of individuals documented the slow destruction of the Kirkbride and its outlying buildings. Outside of official walkthroughs, John Archer endeavored to take as many photographs of the hospital as he could, including the previous iconic shot of the abandoned Kirkbride with a visitor's bench getting lost in the overgrowth. Archer was one of the last people inside of the Kirkbride, photographing the building as it shook from the impact of demolition. Also pictured is one of the wing spires similar to the one that Archer would later add to his home in Danvers. (John Archer.)

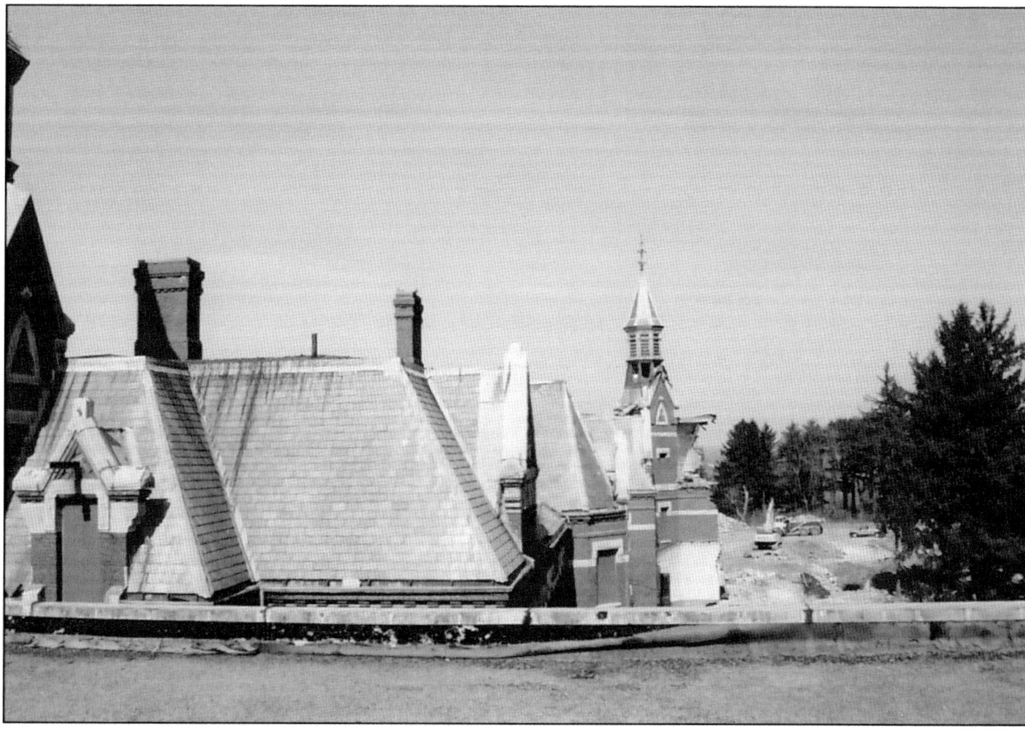

Another often photographed architectural feature of the abandoned asylum was the stepped back roofline with its copper spires and weathervanes decorated with dahlias, the Victorian symbol for madness. The slate roofs survived long enough to be stripped for salvage as demolition began. A portion of that roofline still exists, crowning the new construction at Halstead Danvers. In a letter to the editor of a Danvers newspaper, John Archer wrote, "I have no illusions that AvalonBay's creations will stand the test of time as did the Kirkbride." Two of the wrought-iron spires salvaged from the wing towers now reside with Archer. (Both, John Archer.)

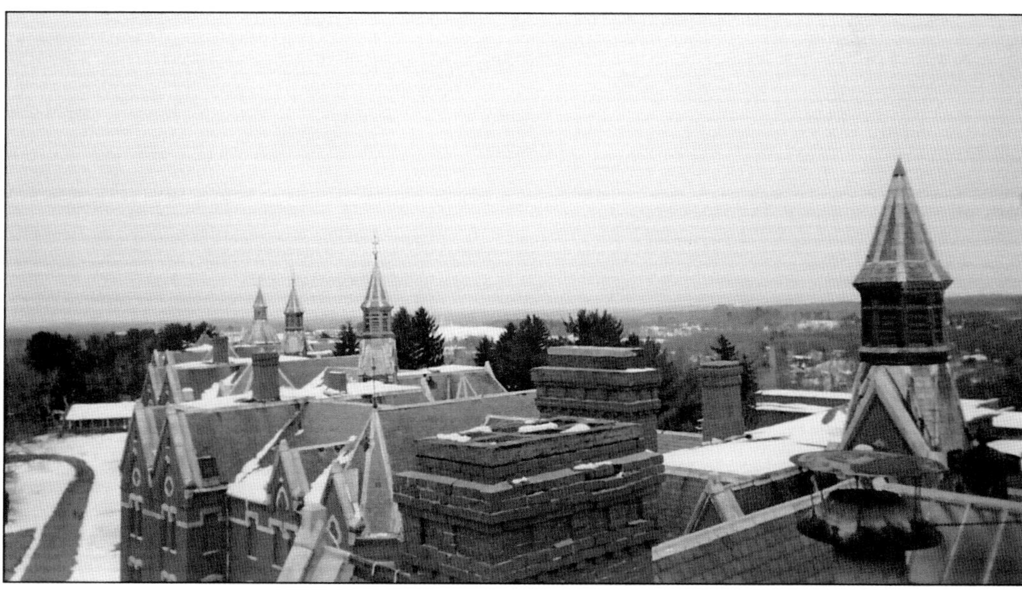

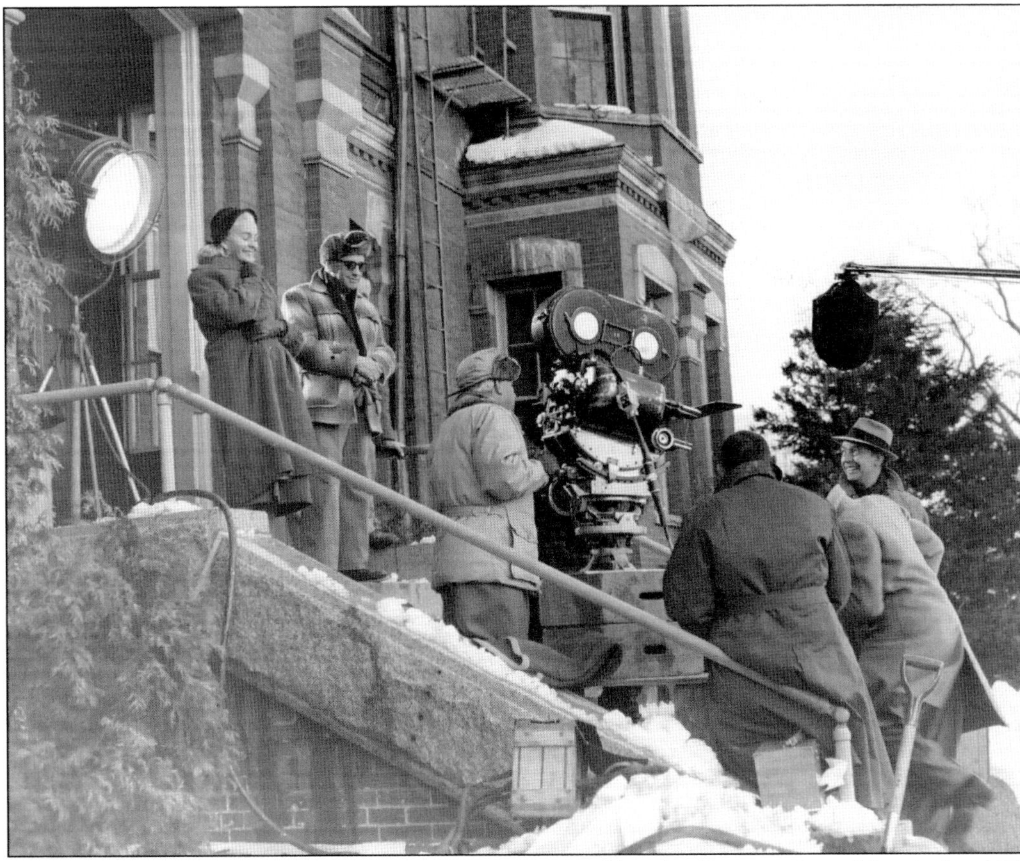

Home Before Dark, a drama starring Jean Simmons, was filmed at Danvers State Hospital in 1958 when the hospital was still in operation. The film features the winding tree-lined drive up to the main administration as well as the reception area of the asylum. A second movie, *Session 9*, was released in 2001 long after the building had been abandoned. Though the hospital was left largely in its natural state for the movie, the *Session 9* room was staged for filming with photographs and magazine clippings affixed to the wall of a patient room. (Above, Danvers Archival Center, Danvers, Massachusetts; below, John Gray.)

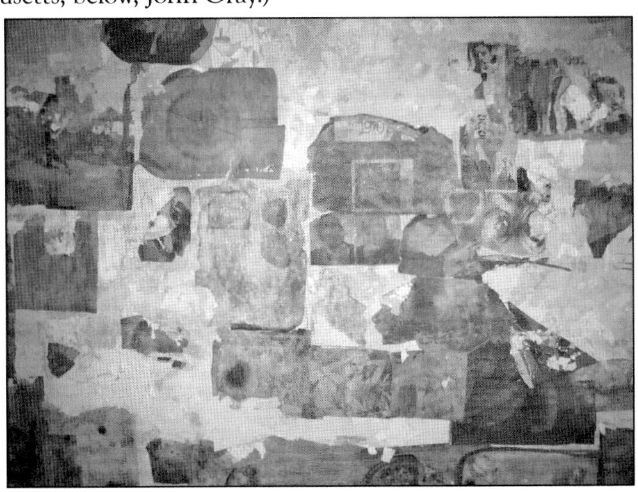

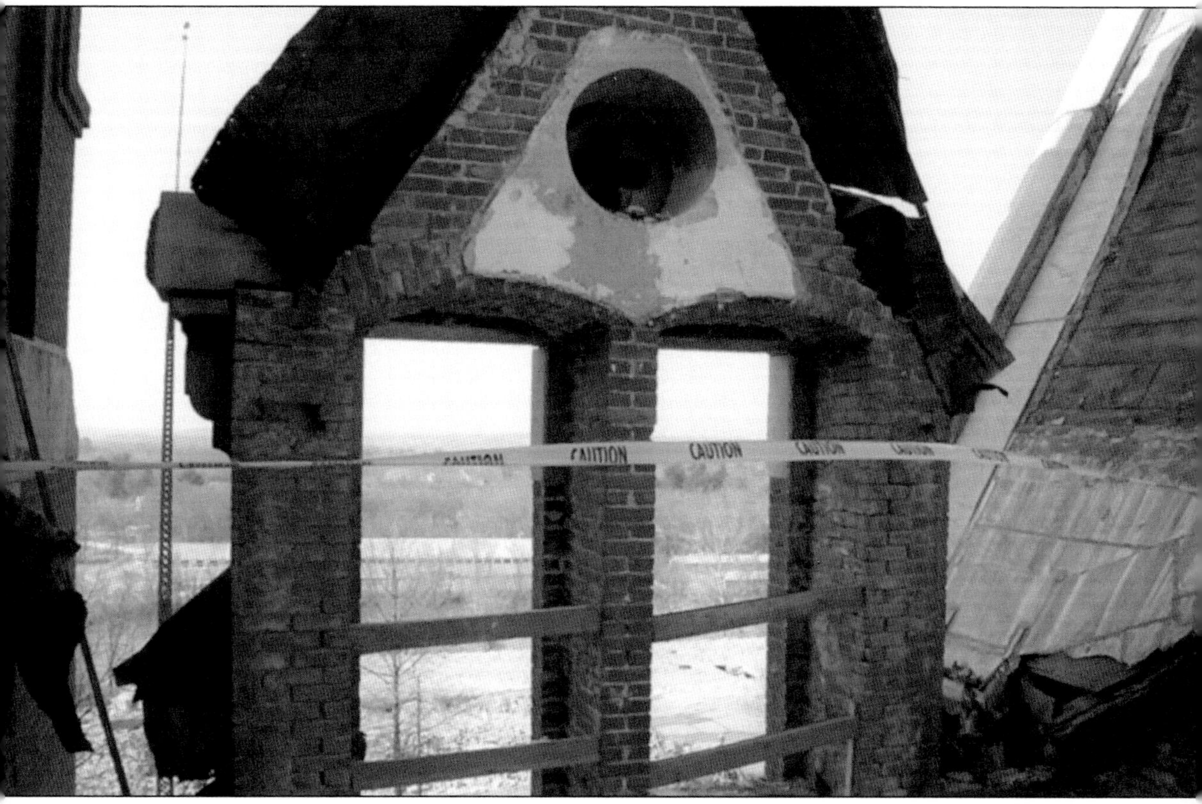

As the battle over the Kirkbride raged, those on both sides of the debate took to the news to air their grievances. For as many preservationists who weighed in, there was an equal number of voices who claimed the asylum was not worth saving, including resident Warren O. Berry, who claimed that the land was increasingly valuable, while the "bricks and mortar" were not. (John Gray.)

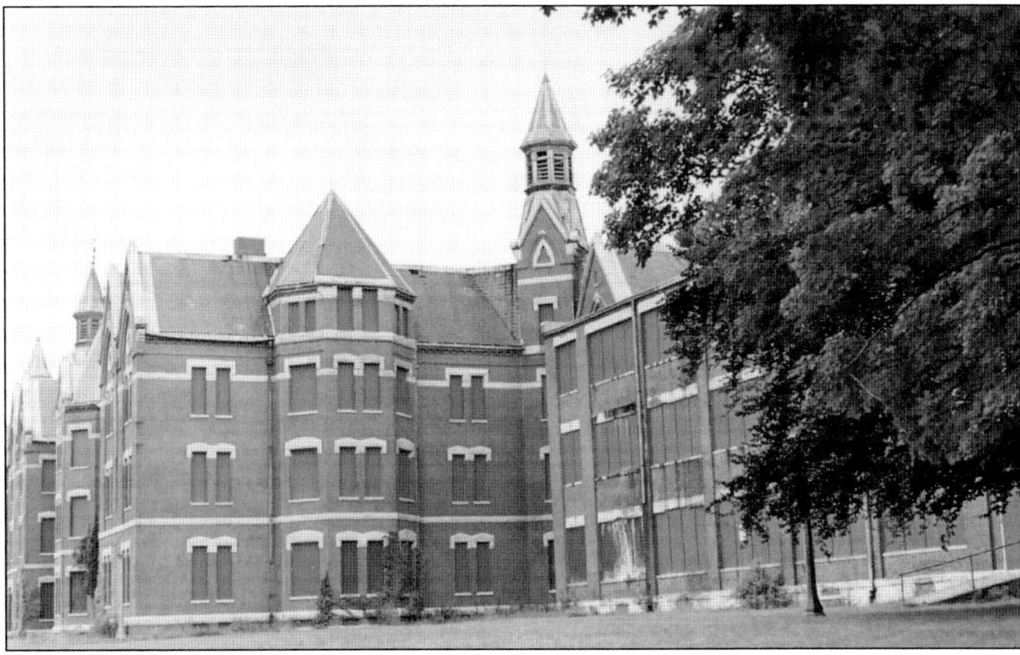

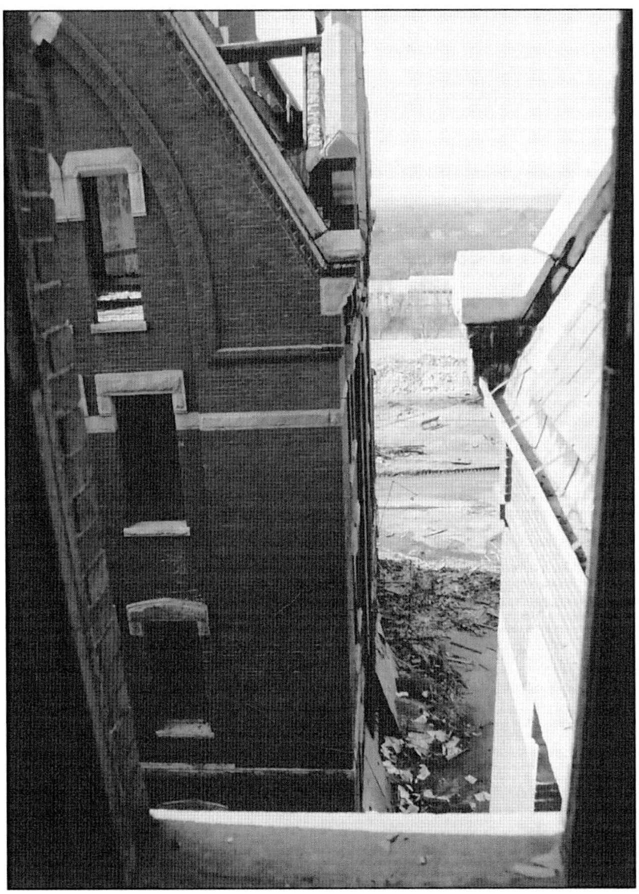

In a July 8, 2002, letter to the editor of the *Salem Evening News* from John Archer, he stated, "We have an opportunity to preserve a unique treasure in the Kirkbride building on the grounds of the former Danvers State Hospital. There is no argument that many terrible things happened during its use as a mental hospital, mostly because of the archaic methods of treatment in use at that time. However, we must not make the mistake of thinking that two wrongs will make a 'right' and that by demolishing the Kirkbride we will exorcise the spirits of those deeply wronged in that institution. . . . Let us not regret its loss in 25 or 50 years' time." (Both, John Archer.)

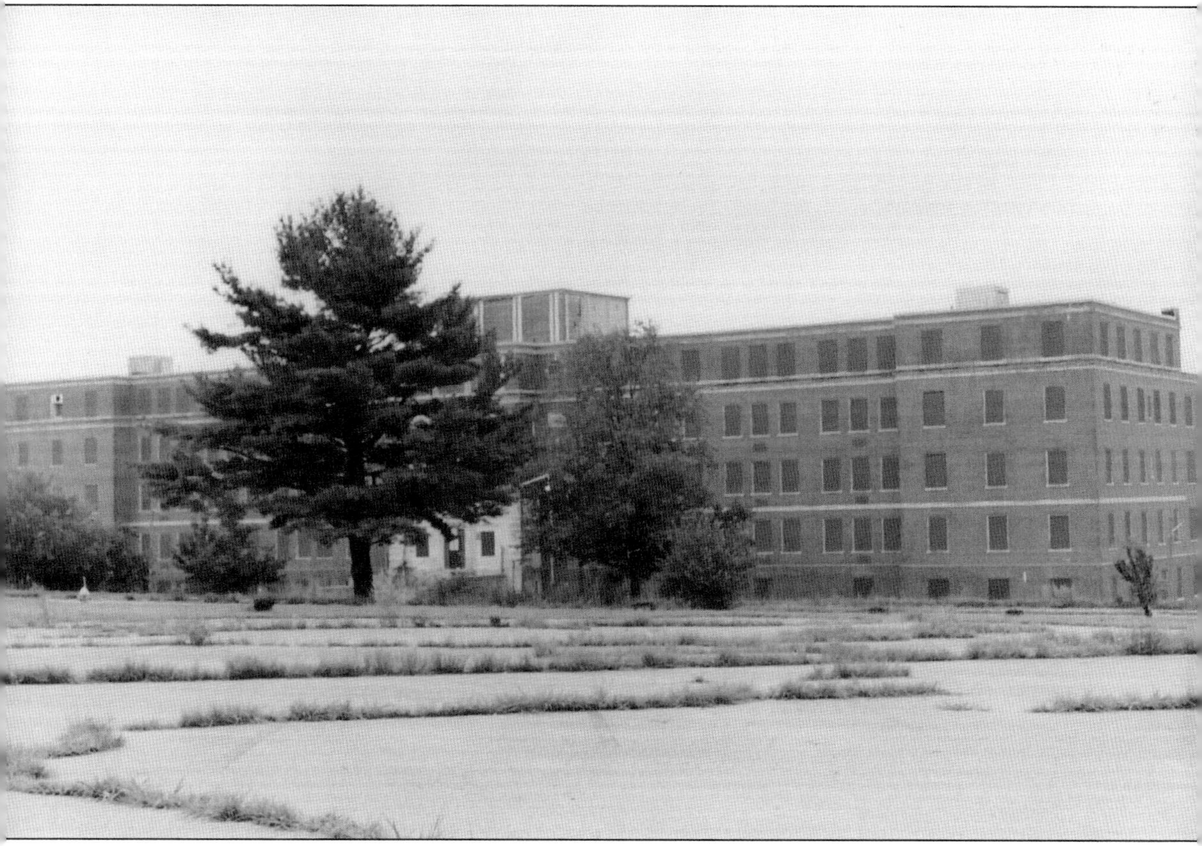

The Bonner Building, once considered a cutting-edge facility for the treatment of the mentally ill, was one of the first buildings to be demolished after AvalonBay took ownership of the property. The sixth floor of the Bonner Building had been converted into a space for a Department of Youth Services program. The morgue was housed on the first floor with an eight-drawer freezer unit. The doors were locked on June 24, 1992. (John Archer.)

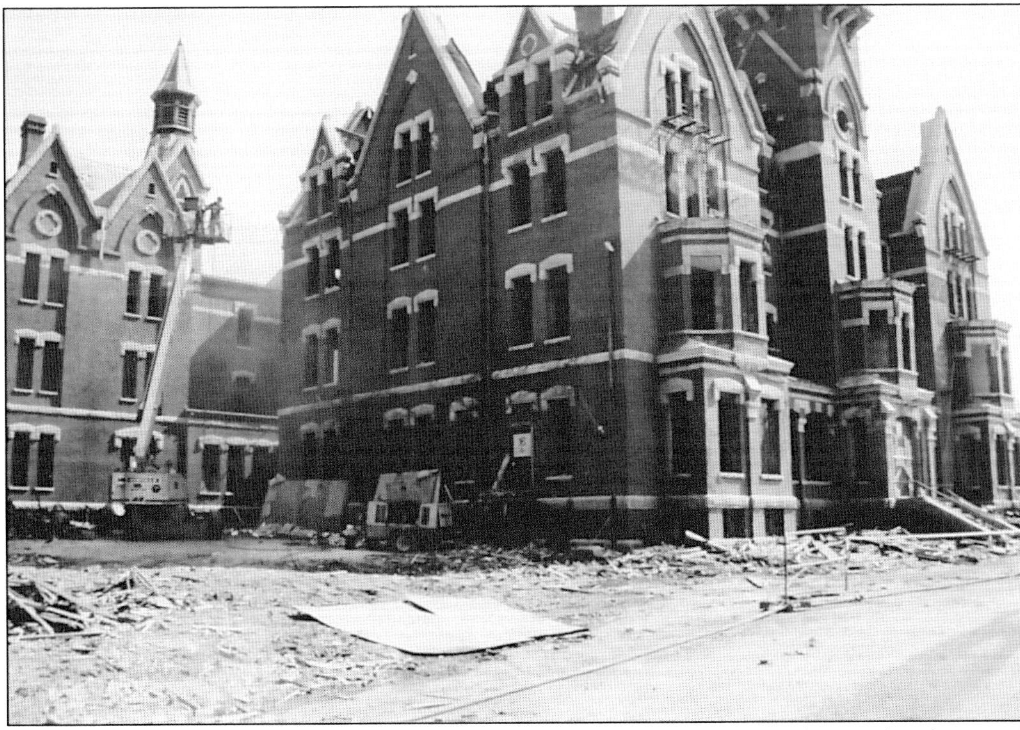

In a December 2005 letter to the editor of the *Salem Evening News* from John Archer, he stated, "I write to you today with a great sadness about the loss of the Kirkbride Building on the grounds of Danvers State Hospital. Despite every effort to preserve this national historic treasure, despite its unique place in the history of the area and in the humane treatment of the mentally ill . . . despite the existence of countless and much older buildings in other parts of the world, the Kirkbride has fallen, a victim of shortsightedness and greed. As I write this letter, the backhoes and bulldozers and wrecking balls are gnawing away at one of the most remarkable architectural treasures of the modern era. I have no illusions that AvalonBay's creations will stand the test of time as did the Kirkbride. In 100 or 500 years, when future historians shake their heads over this tragic mistake, let it be remembered that there were those who had a vision of preservation and reuse of the Danvers State Hospital properties that did not require demolition and cookie-cutter concrete construction. We remember, and so will they!" (Both, John Archer.)

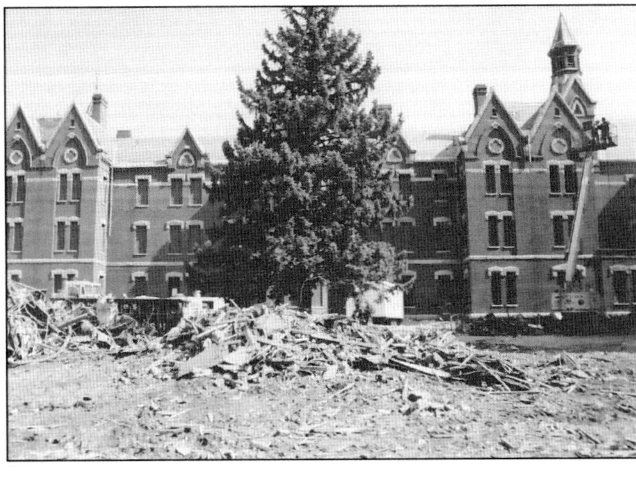

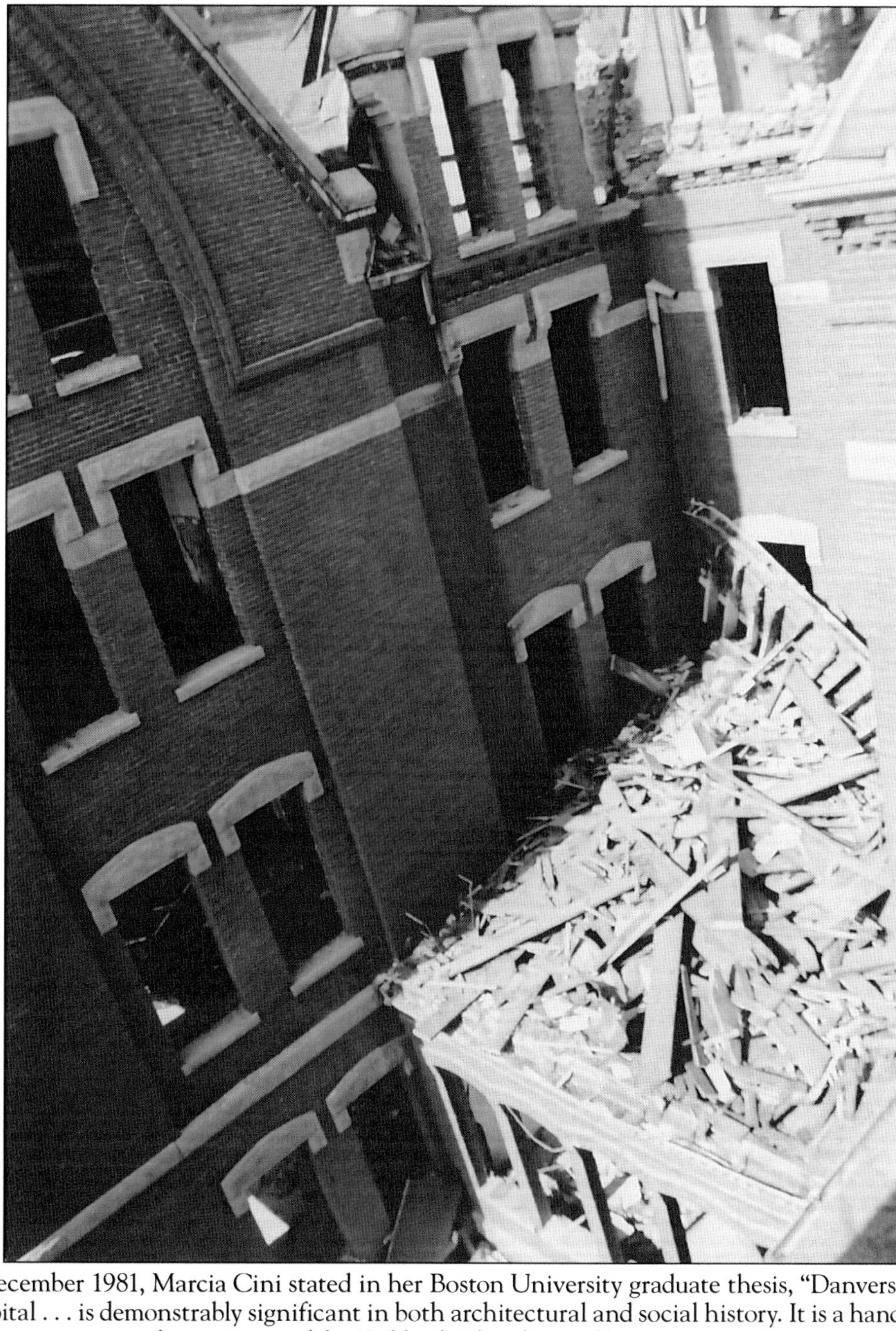

In December 1981, Marcia Cini stated in her Boston University graduate thesis, "Danvers State Hospital . . . is demonstrably significant in both architectural and social history. It is a handsome and uncommon implementation of the Kirkbride Plan directed by an important Boston architect. When built it represented the latest contemporary advances in technology and engineering as well as architecture. Further, its contributions to the history of mental health in Massachusetts are clear. Its current value as an historical resource is increased by the high degree of survival of important original and/or early buildings and the substantial preservation of the original landscape pattern . . . it should be given the protection of listing on the National Register of Historic Places as promptly as possible." (John Archer.)

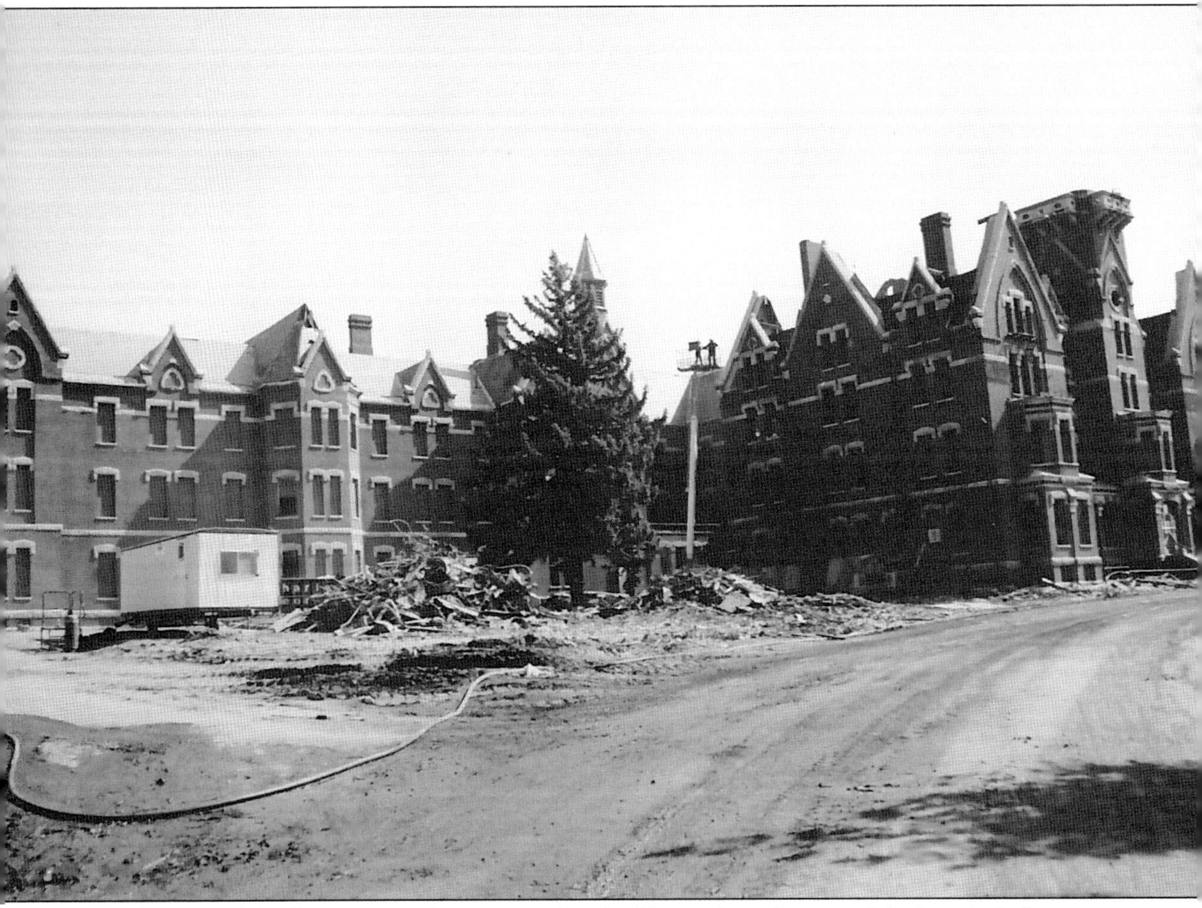

In the late 1980s, the position of superintendent had been phased out, and the hospital closure was overseen by an assistant superintendent. Despite the certification of the Kirkbride as a national landmark and its addition to the Federal National Register of Historic Places, the building was gutted, and all of its outbuildings were destroyed, including the surgery building, Gray Gables, the nurses' quarters, and what remained of the farm. Only the Hogan Regional Center remained standing and in operation. At the foot of the hill now stands the Lahey Outpatient Center formerly known as the Beverly Hospital at Danvers. (John Archer.)

Five

Echoes

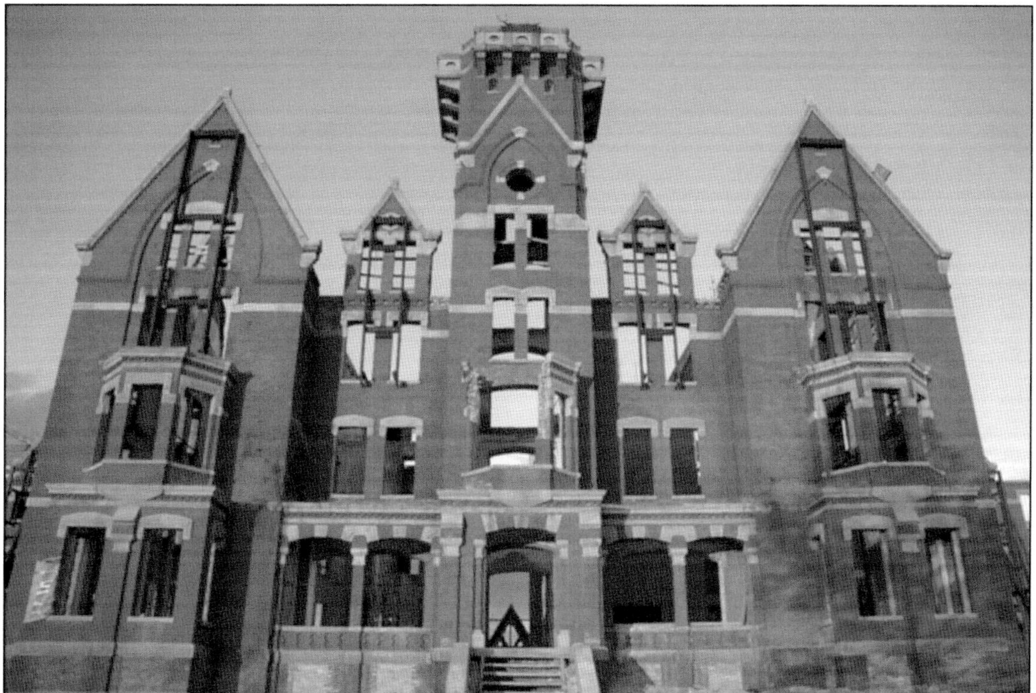

In October 2005, the Danvers Preservation Fund filed an injunction to prevent AvalonBay from moving forward with demolition. Unfortunately, the temporary restraining order was denied and demolition began. The only thing that was retained was the shell of the Kirkbride, shown here stripped of all but the brick façade. (John Gray.)

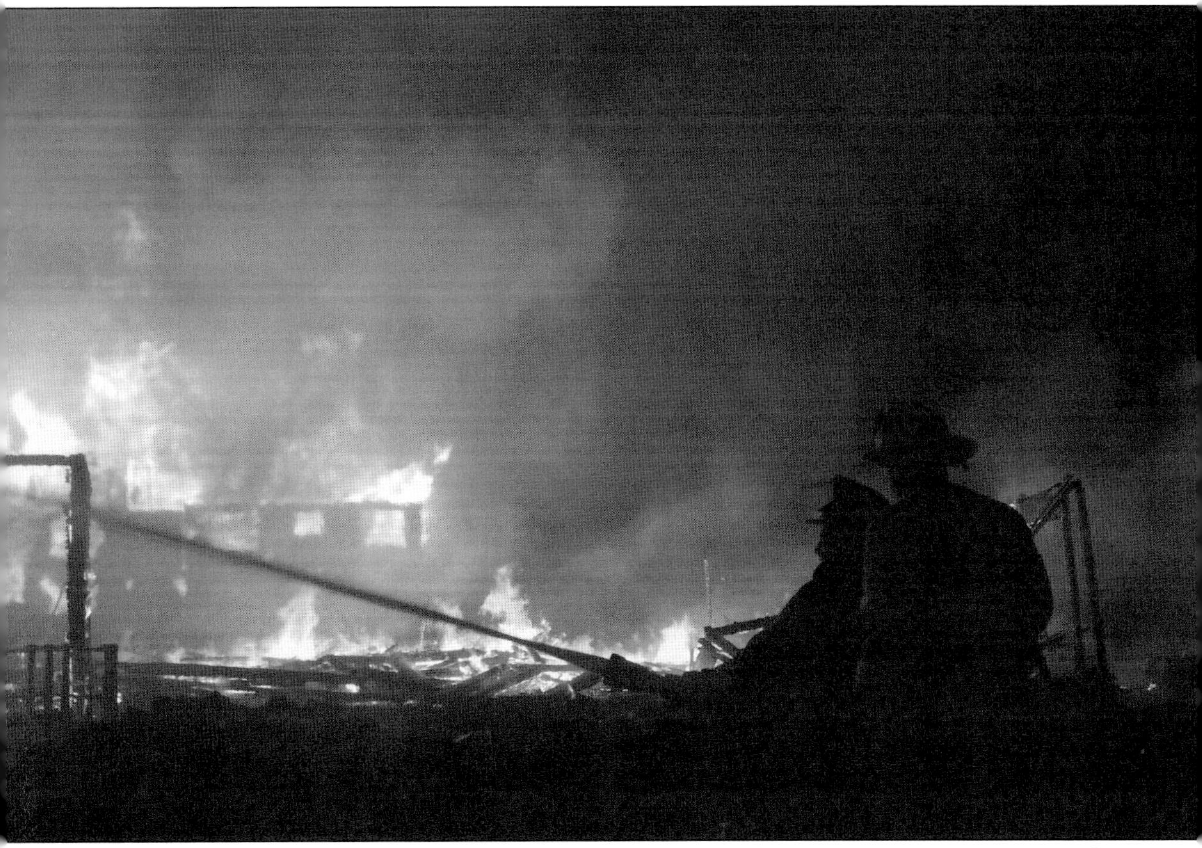

At 1:50 a.m. on April 7, 2007, a four-alarm fire ripped through the new construction at Avalon Danvers, destroying four apartment buildings and damaging one of the cupolas that was being refurbished. Crews from eight surrounding towns responded to the fire and continued to battle the flames that could be seen from the highway well after sunrise, but the buildings were reduced to rubble. All that remained of the 147 apartments were the towers of concrete that encased the stairwells and elevator shafts. A number of apartments on the other side of the property were already occupied, and all 20 residents were evacuated. (John Duffill.)

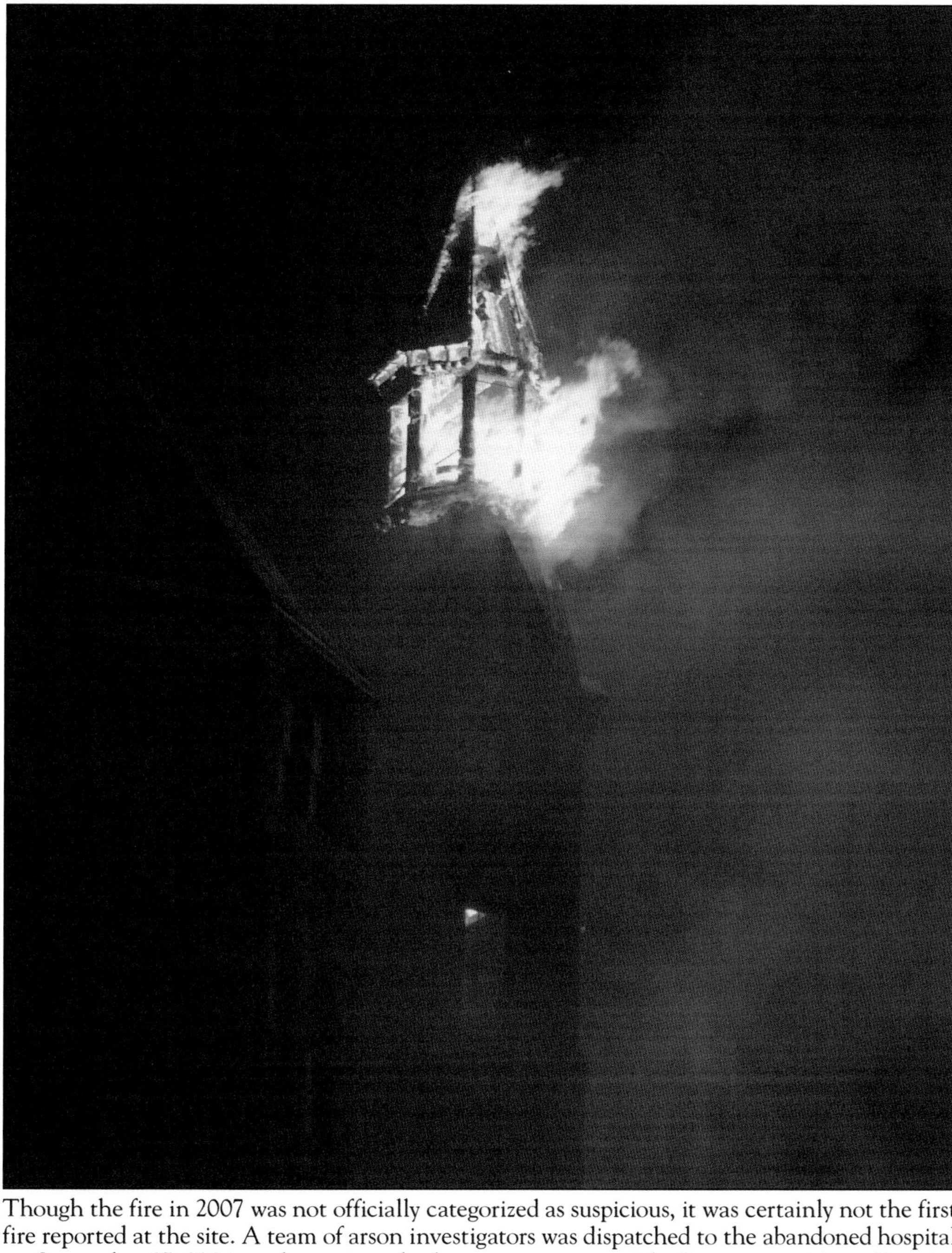

Though the fire in 2007 was not officially categorized as suspicious, it was certainly not the first fire reported at the site. A team of arson investigators was dispatched to the abandoned hospital on September 27, 2004, to determine whether or not an overnight fire was suspicious. Security guards reported smoke the night before, with the fire having started in a pile of old files on the second floor of the main Kirkbride, which luckily was contained within a small hallway on the second floor of the building. Firefighters were able to knock down the flames in minutes, but the already-deteriorated building made for a dangerous situation. The fire had been smoldering for some time before breaking, likely caused by someone discarding a cigarette while exploring; however, the possibility still remained that it was set on purpose. (John Duffill.)

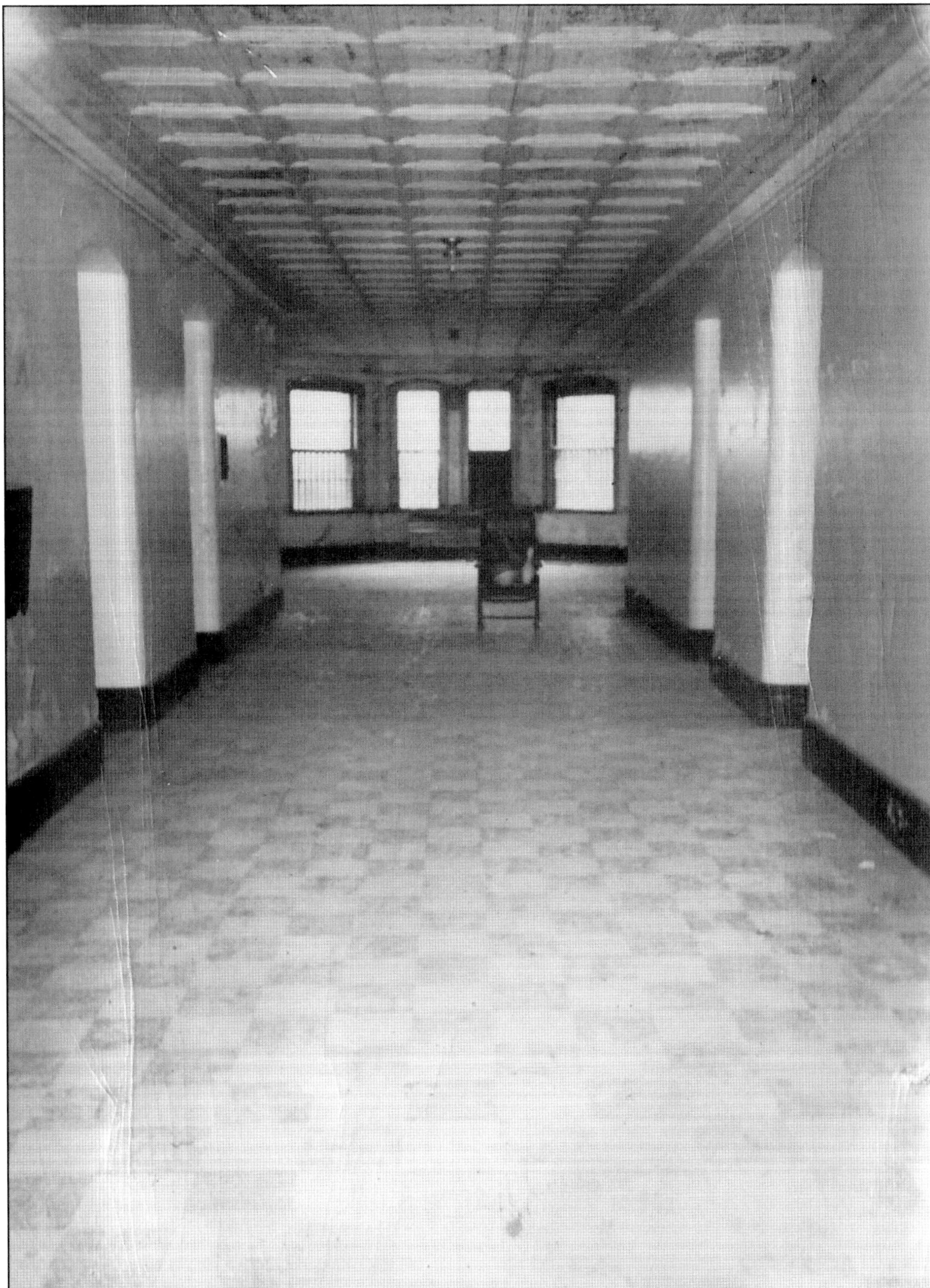

Sculptor A. Andrew Chulyk, a former employee of Danvers State Hospital, created a series of sculptures utilizing bits and pieces of everyday items found on the wards before and after the hospital's closure. This photograph was included as part of one of the installations, attached to a cafeteria tray that rested on the seat of the chair pictured here. (Robert Duffy.)

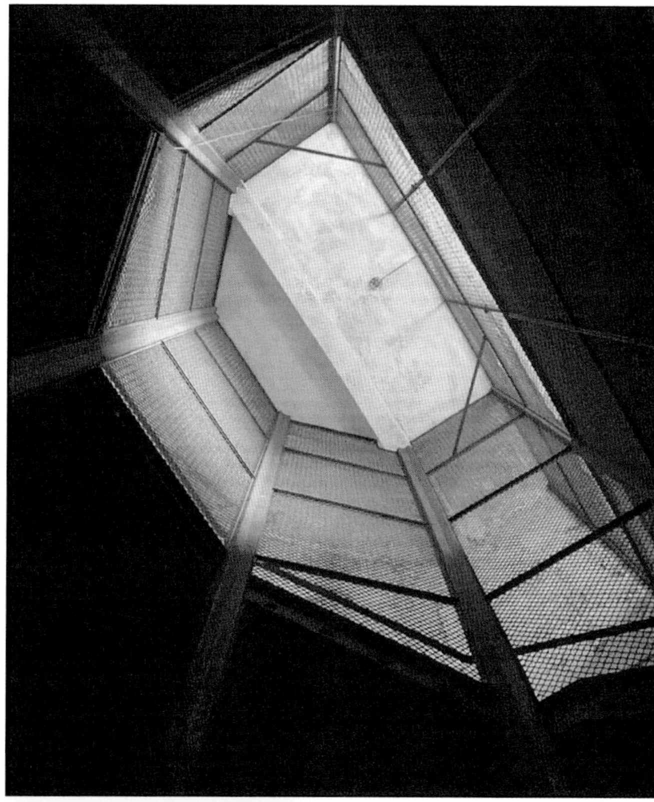

As the Kirkbride was dismantled, much of the salvaged material was transferred to Nor'east Architectural Salvage in South Hampton, New Hampshire. Windows, doors, doorknobs, and door plates were collected and multiple loads of brick were removed from the demolished wards. The metal staircases that had early on replaced the hand-carved wooden stairwells were removed and scrapped. Other pieces such as scraps of decorative tin, light fixtures, and patient room doors were delivered to John Archer's home in Danvers. The tunnels that connected the entire campus were sealed off and, in some cases, dug out and removed. (Both, John Gray.)

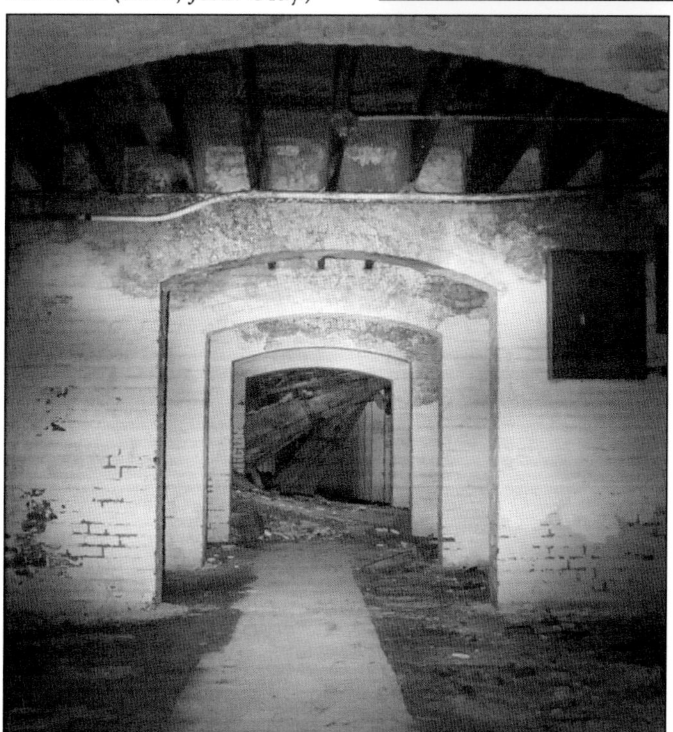

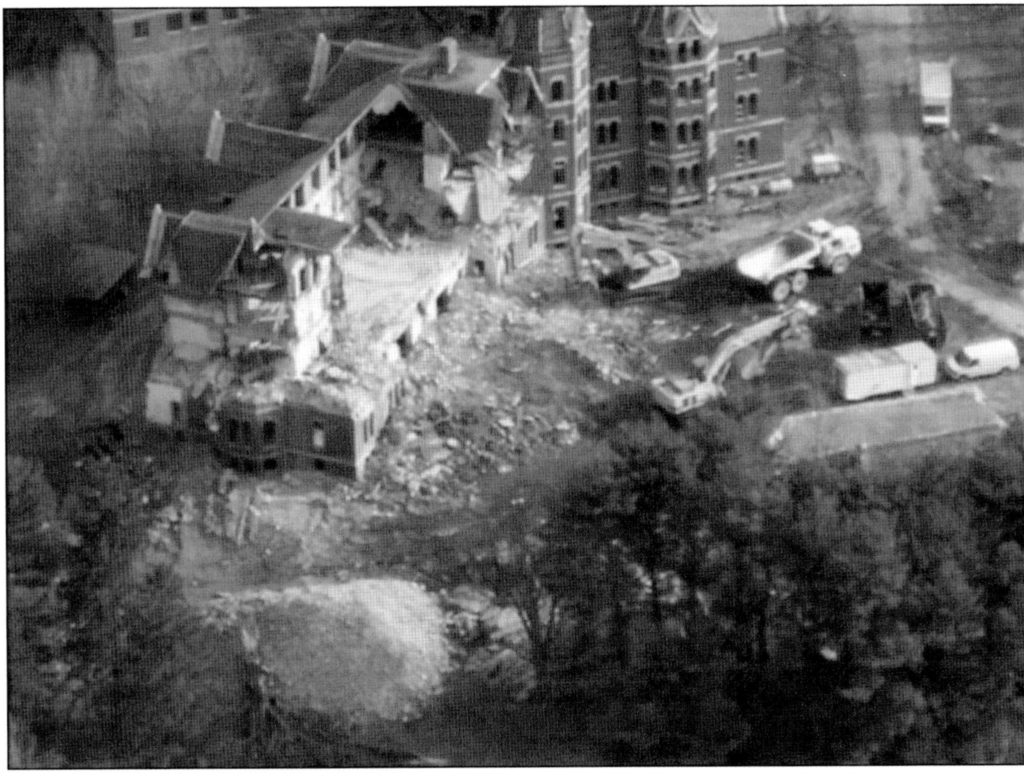

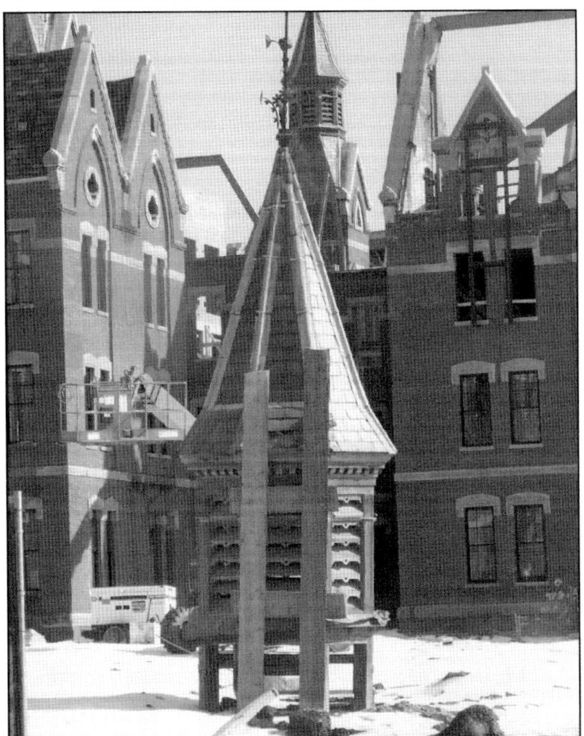

On January 6, 2006, abatement began at the Kirkbride on Hathorne Hill. Above is an aerial image taken by Kim Albright of Abandoned but Not Forgotten showing the hollowing out of one of the hospital's furthermost wards. The hinged wards, A and J, housed the "extreme" or excited patients and were the most unique architectural features of Danvers State Hospital. The spires were removed, some of them retained and reused on the new construction. The superior craftsmanship of Danvers State Hospital was dismantled quickly; demolition was completed in the space of five months, with Ward C being demolished on June 14, 2006. (Both, Kim Albright.)

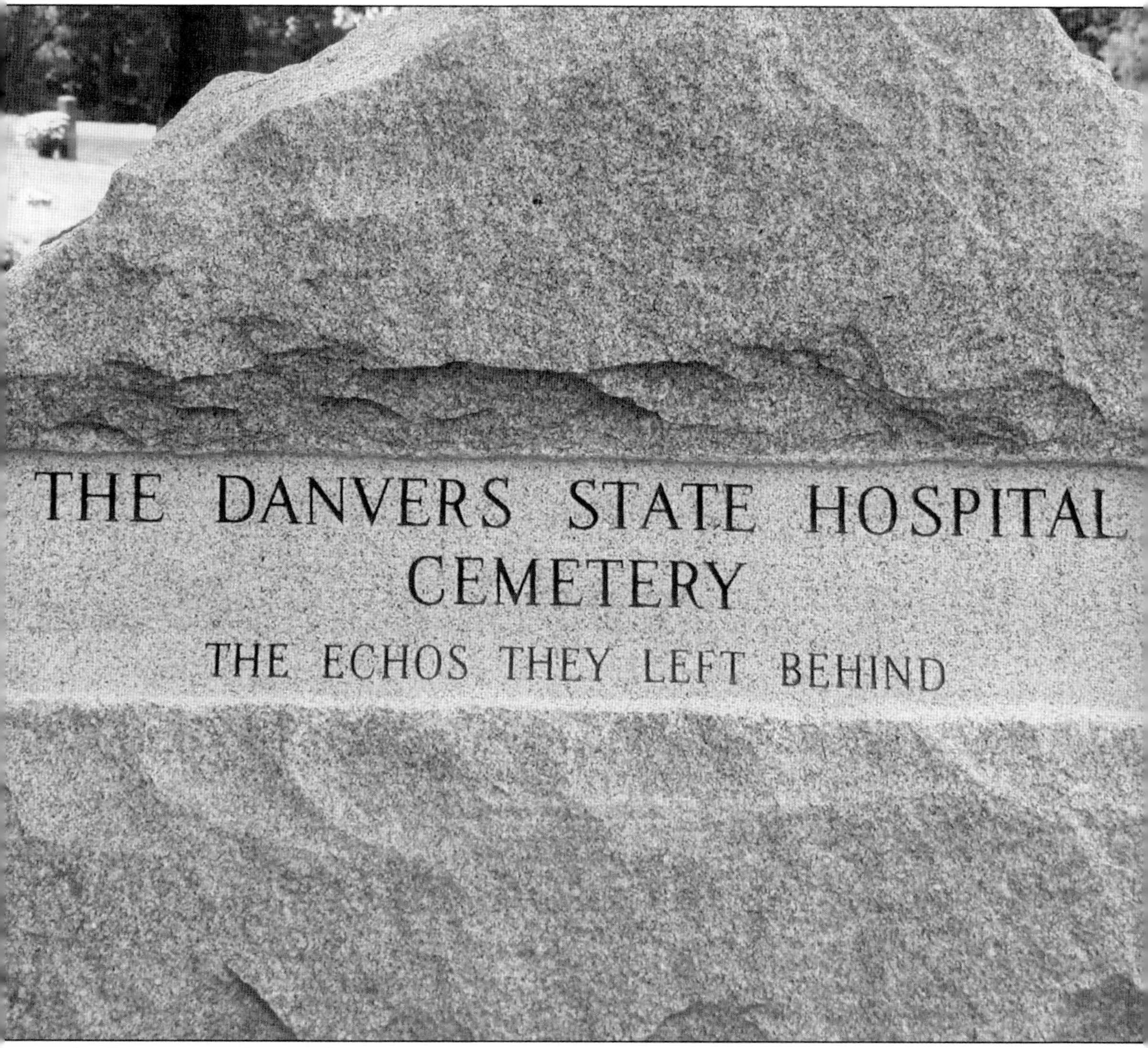
THE DANVERS STATE HOSPITAL
CEMETERY
THE ECHOS THEY LEFT BEHIND
At the opening of a secluded hill surrounded by trees sits the north cemetery, largely forgotten and unmarked, except for this engraved boulder tucked into the mouth of the cemetery. The entrance is located down a steep gravel path behind a private residence, across the road from a long block of condominiums. Inside, a list of the patients whose graves were identified is engraved on a large black stone, with a bench set next to it. The grave markers are arranged in chronological order up to 1906 at the top of the hill, with 1926 into the 1950s at the bottom of the hill. There is a 20-year gap in the stones, only some of which have been identified. The Danvers State Memorial Committee worked to identify as many of the patients as possible so that the cemetery would be "at least as dignified as a pet cemetery." (John Gray.)

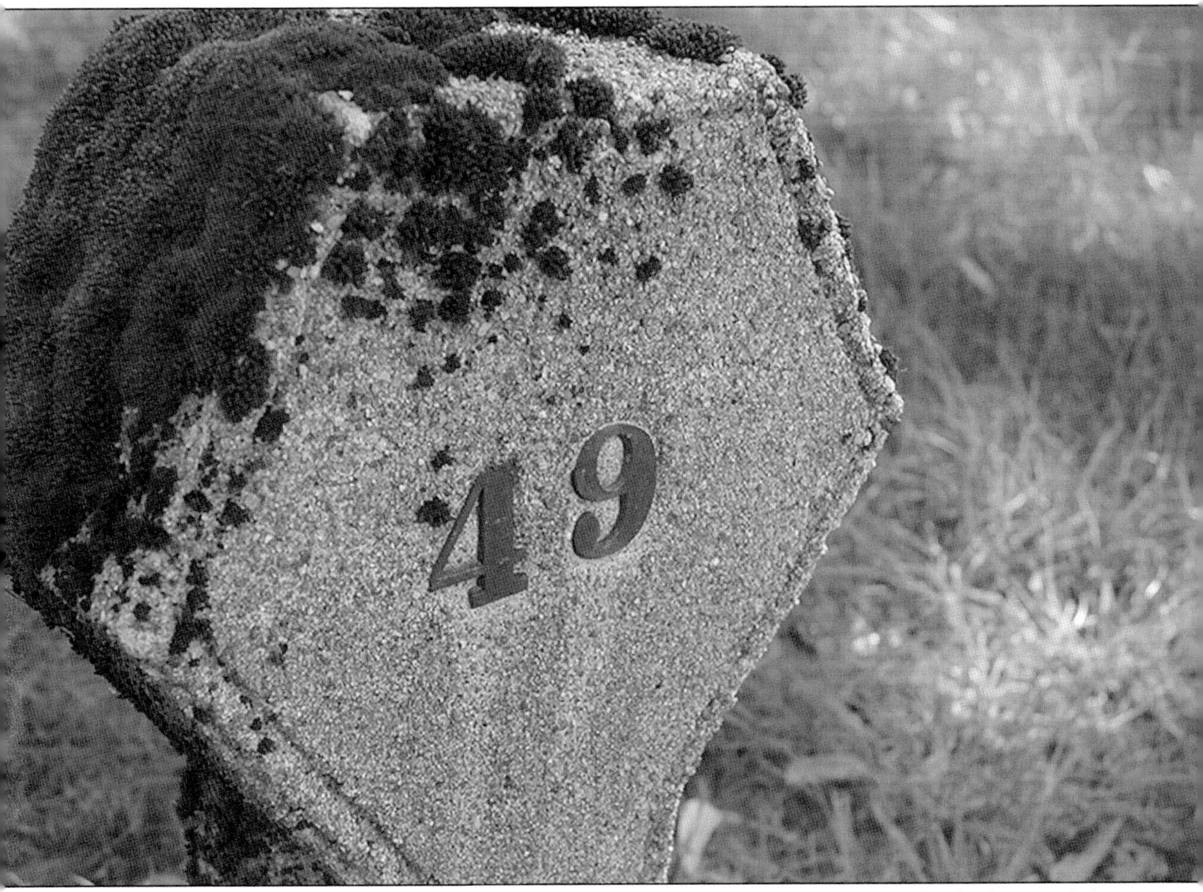

When patients were buried at the state hospital, families rarely came to claim the bodies, and they were buried on the property under numbered markers, such as this one. The headstone is made of molded stone, and the numbers are copper pressed into the stone. Many of these headstones remained the only identification for hundreds of years until a local woman stumbled on the unkempt cemetery while walking her dog and reported it to authorities. The process by which the graves were identified was a long and often difficult search through records that were often missing or incomplete. (John Gray.)

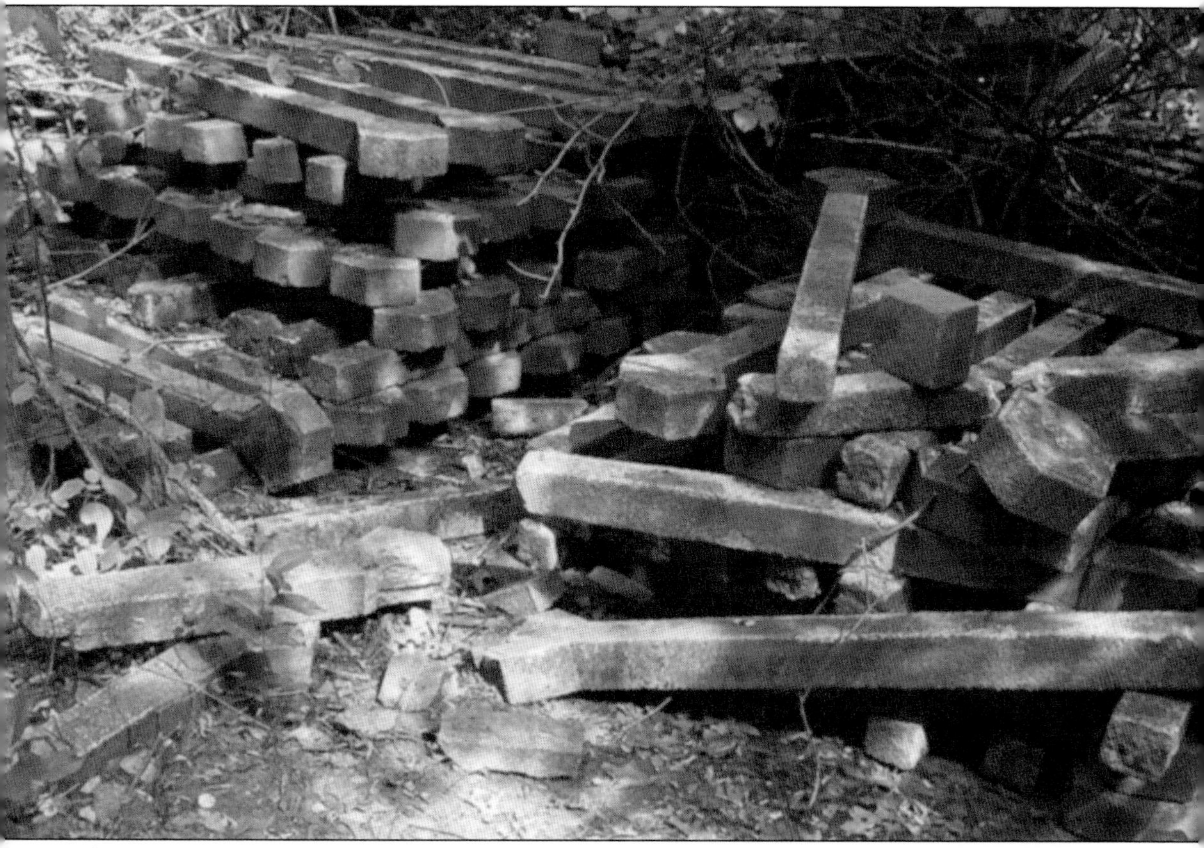

There are two cemeteries dedicated to Danvers State Hospital patients. The north cemetery is located on what is referred to as the "highlands" of the state hospital campus, now situated behind new construction. The south cemetery is located near the former Middleton Farm Colony. There are 770 graves between both sites; the north cemetery has 677 people buried, with 542 identified and 354 have matching nameplates along with their number. The south cemetery has 93 numbered markers with 84 identified, but the names could not be matched with the numbers. This smaller cemetery features the iconic pentagonal headstones pictured here. (Both, John Gray.)

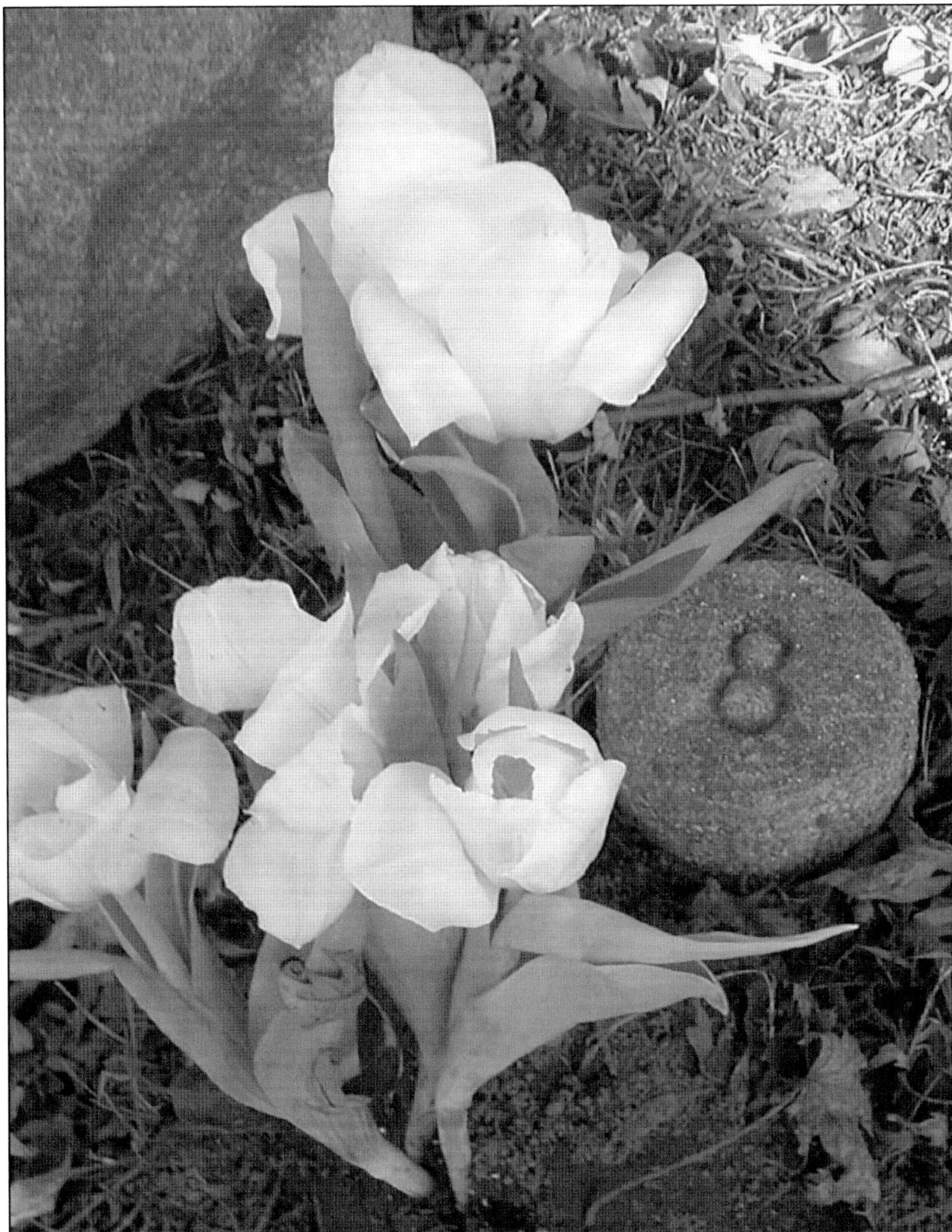

In 2003, photographer John Gray, along with Kristen Polci-Parsons, Dave Walsh, and Christopher Sparks, quietly planted tulips on the graves in the north cemetery. The tulips, which were donated by artist Anna Schuliet-Haber, had been used in an interactive art installation called "Bloom." Schuliet-Haber laid thousands of flowers throughout the wards of Massachusetts Mental Health Center to honor former state hospital patients. She completed a similar installation at Northampton State Hospital, wiring the building to play Bach's *Magnificat*. After "Bloom" was dismantled, Schuliet-Haber began donating the flowers to the few state hospitals still in operation. Gray says he immediately thought of Danvers and took the tulips from the artist. The group fondly nicknamed the project "Operation Tiptoe." (John Gray.)

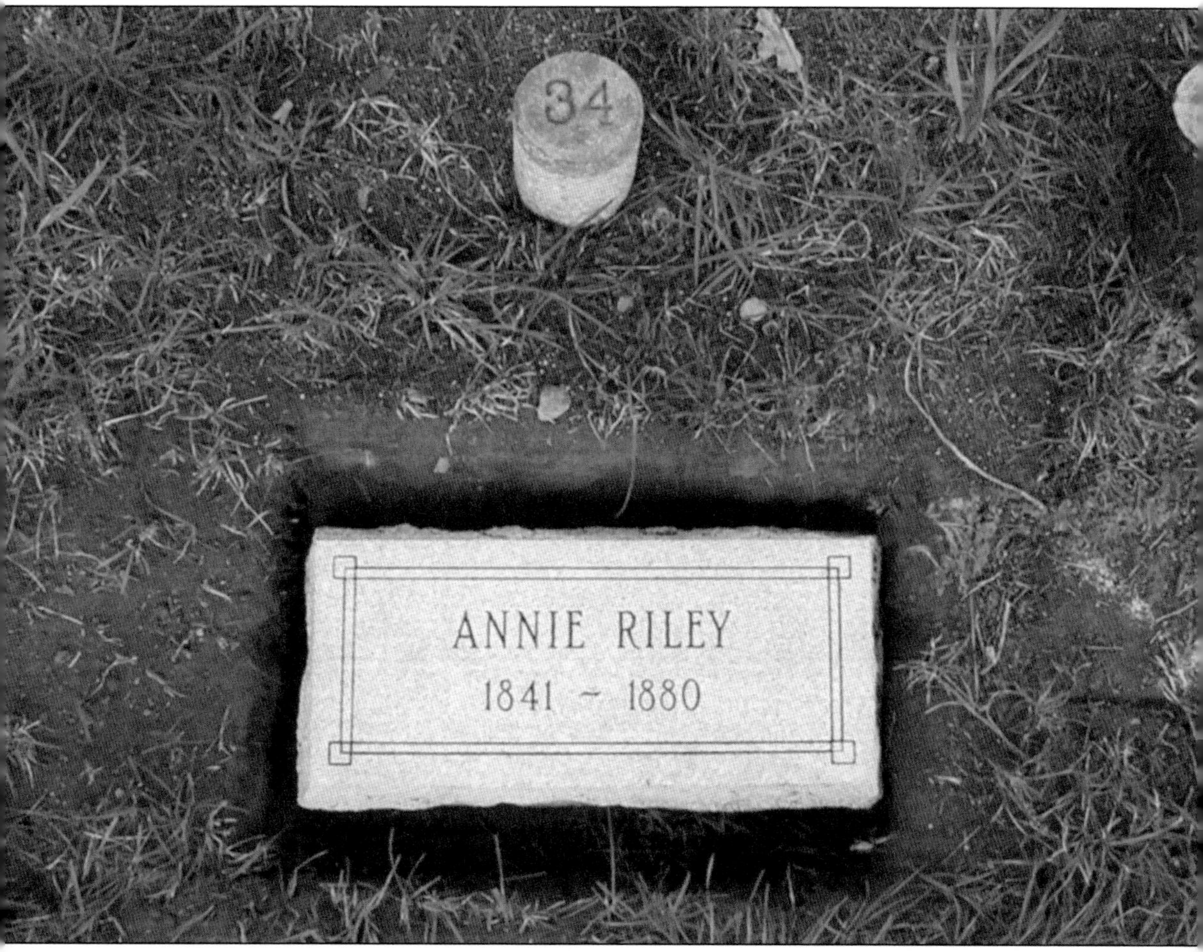

Nearly every state hospital in the United States has a similar cemetery marked only by rows and rows of small, numbered concrete markers, very few of them linked to actual patient names. In 1997, a local resident stumbled on the unmarked cemetery while walking her dog and reported the cemetery's condition, which led to the creation of the Danvers State Memorial Committee. On September 25, 2002, photographer John Gray was invited to document a private ceremony where flowers were planted, and a bell rung as each patient's name was read aloud. Former patients shared their stories, with some wishing the hospital be destroyed while others still admired the architecture and enjoyed seeing it again. (Both, John Gray.)

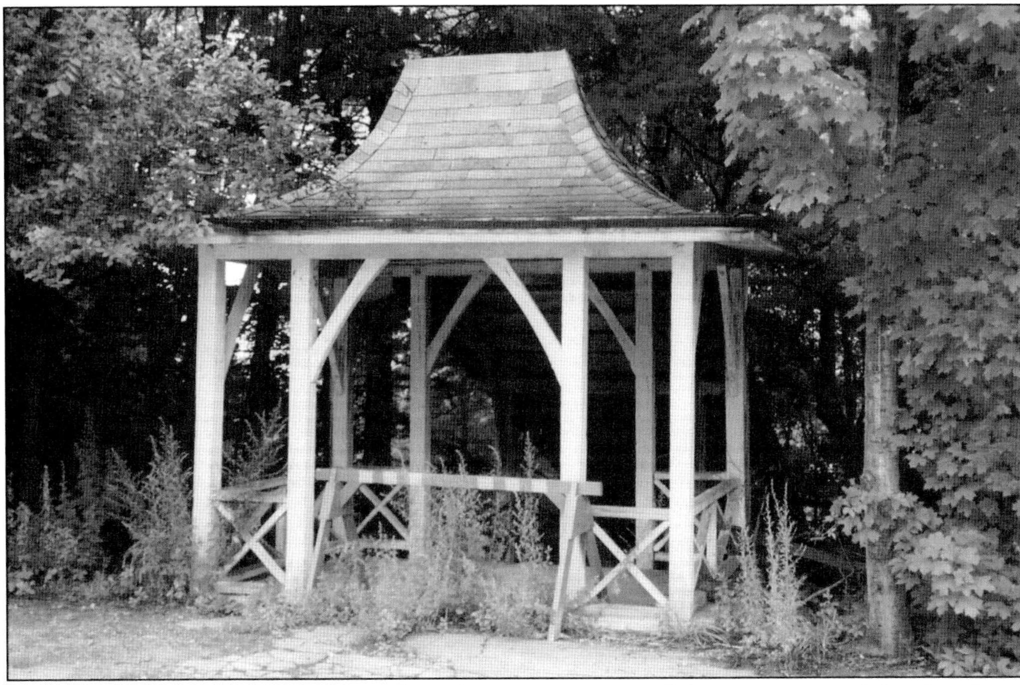

During the filming of *Session 9*, a number of scenes were created that incorporated the abandoned covered staircases at the rear of the Kirkbride. The film shows the characters descending the staircases into a cemetery lined with the tall five-sided gravestones. In reality, those gravestones were located on the lowlands in the south cemetery. The lines of graves and broken gravestones shown in the movie were made of Styrofoam and were added to a field on the highlands side of the Kirkbride in order to create the overgrown, tree covered cemetery in the film. (Above, John Archer; below, John Gray.)

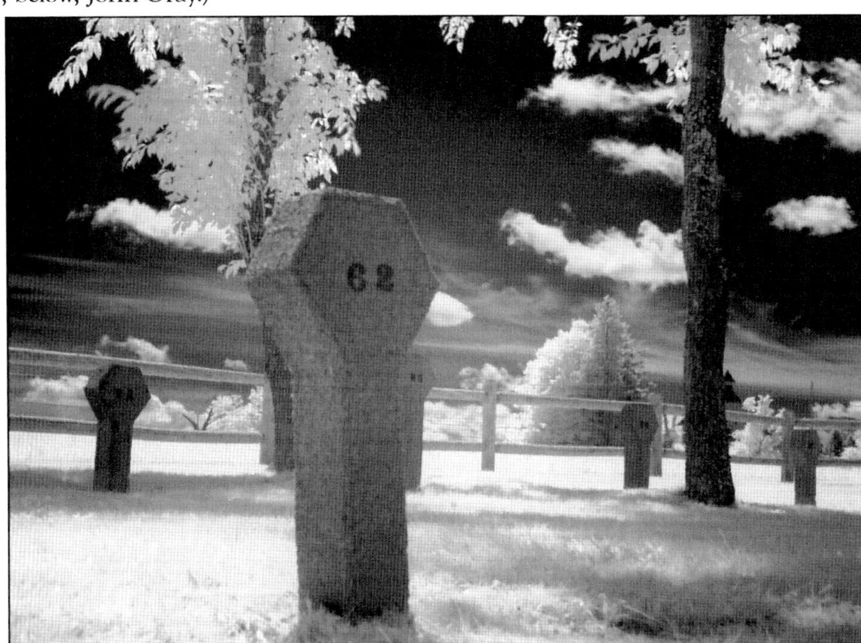

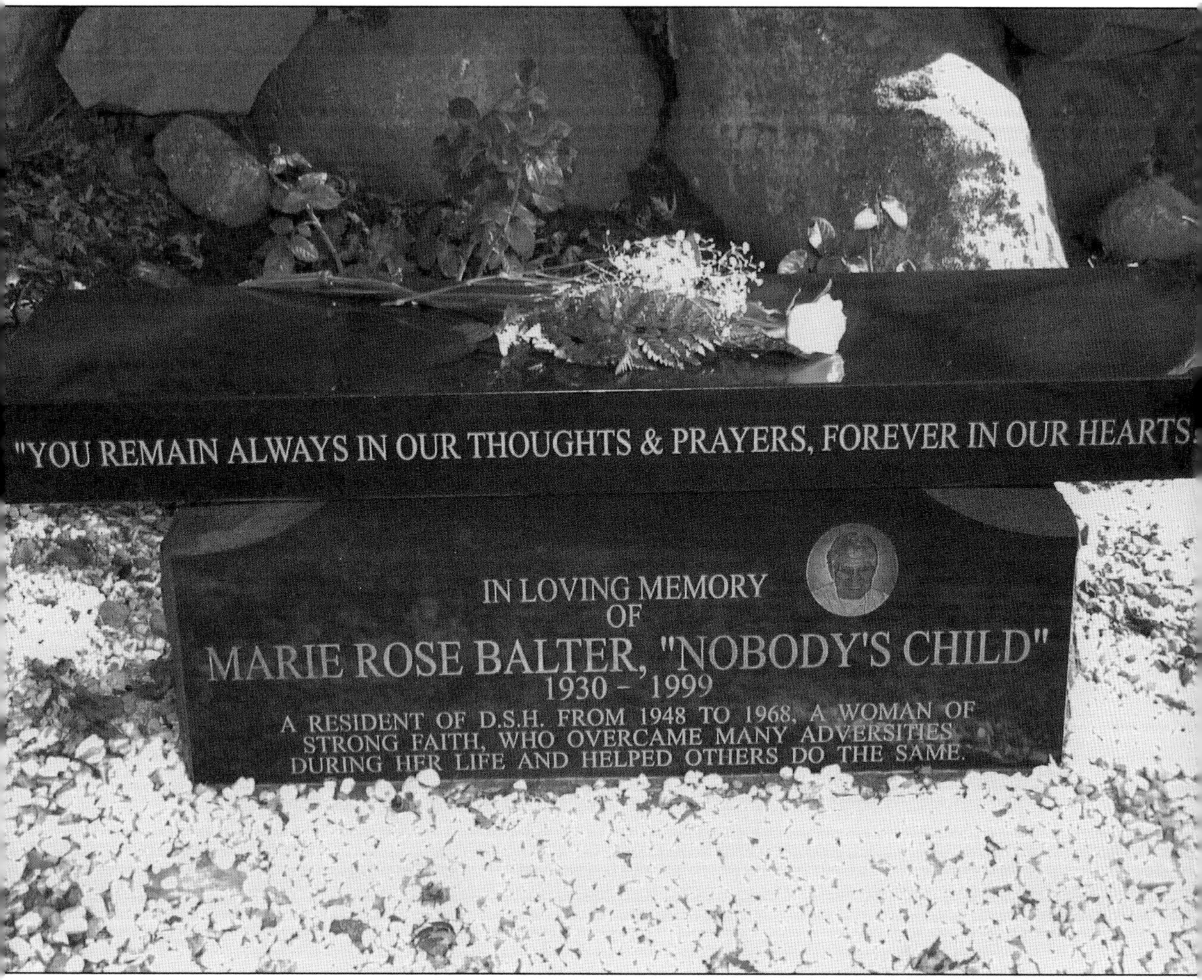
"YOU REMAIN ALWAYS IN OUR THOUGHTS & PRAYERS, FOREVER IN OUR HEARTS."
IN LOVING MEMORY
OF
MARIE ROSE BALTER, "NOBODY'S CHILD"
1930 - 1999
A RESIDENT OF D.S.H. FROM 1948 TO 1968, A WOMAN OF
STRONG FAITH, WHO OVERCAME MANY ADVERSITIES
DURING HER LIFE AND HELPED OTHERS DO THE SAME.

Marie Balter, born in 1931, moved from one foster home to another until she was six years old, when she was adopted by a strict Italian couple who did not speak English. They disciplined her by locking her in the cellar or tying her to a post. She was committed to Danvers State Hospital in the early 1950s and spent 15 years of her life on the locked back wards. Misdiagnosed as schizophrenic, Marie's weight dropped to 86 pounds, and she became catatonic, but when she realized how she had cut herself off from the world, she began to take walks and work on the unit until she was released in 1966. She went on to receive her master's degree from Harvard, returning to Danvers as a hospital administrator. She would later pen a memoir entitled *Nobody's Child*, which detailed her experiences at Danvers. It was later made into a TV film with Marlo Thomas playing Marie. She is memorialized in the state hospital cemetery. (John Gray.)

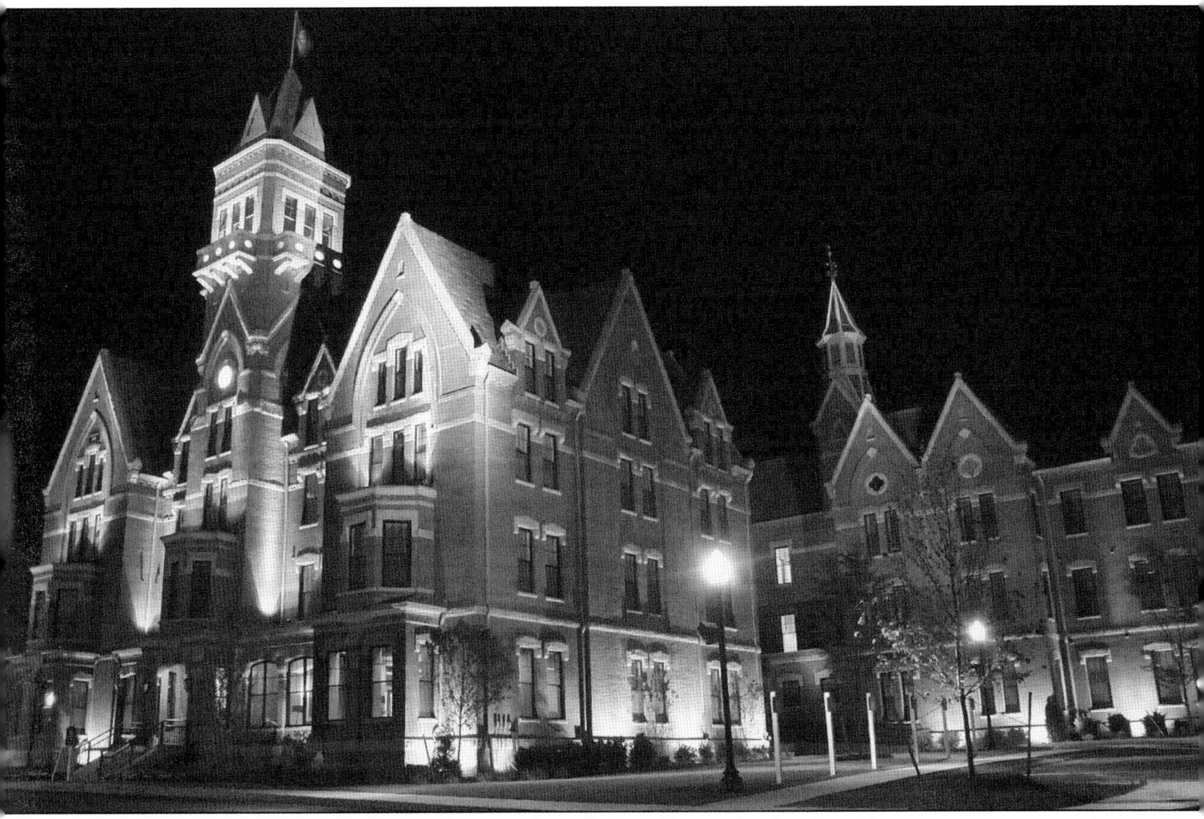

After years of construction and more than $80 million, AvalonBay Communities opened to new tenants in June 2008. Seven years later, the property was purchased by an investment firm and reopened as Halstead Danvers. The 433-apartment complex was transformed into a luxury community offering a state-of-the-art media room, onsite concierge service, and an onsite dog park. Though the shell of the Kirkbride was integrated into the main apartment building, there are no other signs of the asylum that once occupied Hathorne Hill. There is no history provided to tenants, and to date, there is no memorial to the state hospital onsite despite promises from the developer. There is a sitting area overlooking the towns of Danvers and Peabody that the town says will soon have informational plaques, but thus far, the stone ledges remain empty. (John Gray.)

A Tale of Two Hills

Where lie the answers to the architecture of old?
Buried deep in the past where their stories remain untold.
Ancient relics of beauty that once held a dream
Are now structures of emptiness under the suns glaring beam.

How harsh the reality of what once was the past
Where pinnacles of luxury were constructed to last.
Nestled high upon hilltops, unattainable by some.
Stand the testaments of luxury and horrors unknown.

From one extreme to another, of those they did contain,
Are found haunting impressions from the souls that still remain.
Foundations of life through living that no longer must exist
To taunt the weakened mind, of those who can't resist.

Was it the joyful laughter of humanity that echoed down the halls?
Or the giddy sound of insanity trapped within their tattered walls?
What have we created? What purpose do they share?
Are they silhouettes of happier days or shadows of despair?

Annette DeClue

This poem, written by Annette DeClue and given to John Archer, was originally featured in artist Michael Ramseur's book *Haunted Palace*, a combination of historical images and pastel drawings Ramseur himself created after numerous visits to the "castle on the hill." Ramseur described Danvers as "grand in size yet so ominous." It inspired him to paint what he imagined life was like inside: "The building told of a time when people struggling with their minds were put away, and those on the outside shivered at the thought of what was happening *in there*." *Haunted Palace* remains, along with Ramseur's other book *The Eye of Danvers*, two of the most comprehensive tellings of the state hospital's history through both art and historical fact. (John Archer.)